HOT FLASHES
IN A COLD WORLD

MY STRUGGLE TO REMAIN A HUSBAND, A DOCTOR
AND A MAN, IN THE FACE OF PROSTATE CANCER

ALAN ROBERTS, M.D., FACP

Dedication

To Janet,
Who is forever mine, gives me her strength when I am
weak, loves me as I am, travels this too short a life with me,
gives it foreverness, and insists always on total honesty.

To my sister-in-law, Karen Steinberg, and our loving friend
Joanie Hardcastle, who allowed me to share my thoughts,
fears and pain.

With grateful thanks to my good friend, Daniel Rahn, M.D.,
without whom there would be no book, as he urged me to
keep a journal from the beginning of my cancer story.

Some names have been changed in the interest of privacy.

Prologue

May 14, 1999

I am not starting at the beginning; rather, with our second day at the Neely house, located on the fifth floor of the New England Medical Center. This is a live-in facility for patients and family who are undergoing some type of cancer treatment at the medical center. They call me Dr. Roberts, but a cancer patient by any other name....

It was there that my initial treatment was rendered, and where I soon realized the difference between being a physician and being a patient. Janet, my strength and my love, was with me, thank God. We had a one-room efficiency in the Neely House, a residence for patients receiving cancer treatment at the medical center, as well as their families. We lived there for three months.

It was there that I began my journal, which was to evolve into this book. "Hot Flashes in a Cold World," describes my thoughts, feelings and experiences, having and dealing with prostate cancer. If I had to divide my narrative into sections, it would be as follows:

1. Learning I had prostate cancer.
2. Living through the treatment.
3. The aftermath: that is, living with cancer after the initial treatment.
4. Being both a physician and patient.

Being a physician and a patient with cancer places me in the rather unique position of being able to educate others about prostate cancer from the vantage point of a physician who has cancer, and exploring and sharing those emotions common to all cancer patients, many of which are so often not talked about and most often not dealt with. This wearing of two hats, as it were, allows me to relate the dizzying day-by-day rollercoaster of my emotions through the course of diagnosis, treatment and its aftermath. I write not just as a patient but as a physician who is a patient, and about how being a physician adds another dimension to an otherwise not so unusual story; and if, in telling my story, I can help one other person deal a little bit better with his illness, and one other physician deal a little bit better with his cancer patients, then this writing will have served its purpose.

My readers will be all of us since we will, all, at some time, have to deal with a life- threatening illness: its treatment, its consequences, its effect on those friends and families who share the event, and are affected by it in such myriad ways. We will experience how devastating it can be, but also how it can be survived (for however long). I can relate how one person experienced this ordeal; and how that one person, being a physician as well as a patient, can offer his experiences, not only for the benefit of patients and families but for physicians as well, with and without cancer.

Prostate cancer is the most common cancer in men. In the United States in 2007 over 200,000 new cases of prostate cancer were diagnosed, and 27,000 deaths were attributed to prostate cancer. Despite the fact that prostate cancer is the second leading cause of cancer death in men, it causes only 3 percent of all deaths in men. There were approximately 180,000 new cases of prostate cancer in the United States in the year 2000. Physicians represent 0.2456 percent of the total population, which means there were approximately 442 new cases of prostate cancer in physicians in the year 2000. There are 611,028 male physicians in the United States and 227,908 male physicians 50 years old or older. Seven in every 10,000 of these physicians are likely to develop prostate cancer each year.

When a doctor becomes a patient, it is truly a remarkable transition. For me, it was not just a struggle to stay alive, but an opportunity to face my own mortality and to feel what my patients might feel in similar circumstances. Through this most humbling experience, I believe I have become a much better doctor, with a far better understanding of what my patients must feel. Add to that what it is like to be chemically castrate and yet deeply in love, and to put into words what being impotent means, and you have some of the reasons I think my memoir will resonate with others who have gone through, or are going through, what I have experienced.

For this reason, and for the effect "Hot Flashes in a Cold World" may have on how physicians care for their patients—not only those with prostate cancer but with other cancers and other life-threatening illness as well—physicians in the United States and elsewhere will want to read this book, as will every man with prostate cancer, and each of their spouses.

I initially asked a freelance editor to review the journal from which this book was born. Her resulting comments had as much to do with her husband's impotence, caused by his taking large amounts of high blood pressure medicines. Until she read my description of what it was like to be impotent, she had no idea how devastating this could be to her husband, nor how to react herself. She now had a much better understanding of what this must be like for him— as well as a much better understanding of her own feelings—after reading my notes about my impotence. She also commented on how difficult it was to discuss these issues with her husband and how little they were informed of the consequences of the medication. She remarked how unimportant the physicians seemed to think the impotence was in relation to the benefits of the medicine, and how difficult it was for the physicians to comfortably discuss the impotence with them.

I know of no other book that is written by a physician who is himself a patient, and who is willing to lay bare his soul in describing his deepest, most intimate feelings that speak to how the experience of cancer, and the treatment thereof, is such a uniquely personal ordeal— and how poorly understood that ordeal is to the treating physicians.

This, then is my memoir. It describes my personal experience with cancer, as both a physician and patient, through the entire course of my illness: diagnosis; then treatment, with its effects both good and bad; the time after the initial treatment; and, particularly, my emotional response.

Moreover, what I have done is to incorporate into my memoir experiences with family members: their tragedies and their blessings, their courage in facing life's travails. I examine how my cancer is woven through a potpourri of events in other lives—lives that include family, friends and patients—and how there often is a common thread that binds them all.

"Hot Flashes in a Cold World" offers a chronicle of events in my life, with the added insight that comes from my being a physician. It is the story of how my life, as a physician and a man, was forever changed by having prostate cancer. My book gives the reader a day-by-day narrative of my diagnosis and treatment, of the side effects of treatment, and of the impact of this illness—its treatment and its aftermath—on my wife and my marriage. The impotence caused by my treatment permeated my experience every minute of every day, and increased my sensitivity and understanding of what my patients, undergoing similar treatment, were feeling and going through.

I lay bare my soul and share with the reader my deepest, most personal and intimate feelings, day by day, as I attempt to deal with my cancer. I also speak of other family events occurring at the same time—some a blessing and some a tragedy.

This comprehensive description of my emotional roller-coaster ride through it all may prove to be the most important element in my book to all readers who have or may develop prostate cancer. Those readers include husbands, their wives and other family members, and those who care for patients with prostate cancer: physicians and non-physicians. The narrative is interwoven with vignettes of encounters with my former and present patients. And I hope I have shown how this experience of having prostate cancer has made me a much more sensitive physician and human being.

This narrative chronicles the events that occurred from diagnosis, through treatment, and after. Readers will find here my description of my impotence caused by the treatment, and how devastating it was to me, both physically and emotionally. I write about how totally ill-prepared I was for what it would be like to be without testosterone.

In "Hot Flashes in a Cold World," I describe what it is like for a physician to become a patient.

Chapter One
Beginning

Often, it seems life goes from one day to the next with very little change. My life, for instance, was that of an ordinary husband, father and physician, in private practice in internal medicine in a small town in South Florida. After a rather unhappy first marriage, I had met Janet and found, as time passed, a love that I never would have imagined could exist.

Sometimes tragedy and success are intermingled and so it was for me. Tragedy, for me, was losing my 18-year-old daughter from my first marriage in an automobile accident, an accident that occurred when I was separated from my first wife. The pain of that loss was almost life-ending for me as well, but somehow, as many find who suffer such a loss, I found I was able to go on—though never, ever, totally free of the pain of that loss.

And, some time after Lori's death, Janet and I found each other and I found a love I never knew existed. We married, and a new life began for us. Janet was born and raised in Atlanta, Georgia, and lived there, married her first husband and bore two daughters there. After we married, Janet, with her two daughters, Meredith and Paige, came to live in south Florida, and we stayed there until I was offered an associate professorship at the Medical College of Georgia in Augusta, Georgia. Meredith went on to the University of Michigan and then to the University of Georgia Law School, and Paige, after graduating from the University of Wisconsin, received a Masters Degree in social work from the University of Georgia.

Without question, our moving to Augusta was a wonderful move for us. Janet had her mother and one sister, Karen, in Atlanta, another sister Marcia, in Thomaston, Georgia. Moreover, the girls had their Dad there, which made the transition for us all much more meaningful. Our life in Augusta, and my role as physician and now professor—practicing medicine in an academic environment, and teaching medical students and young doctors—was surprisingly without significant stress or strain for me, and remarkably gratifying. It seemed that this was, in many ways, a new beginning, even though I was well into the practice of internal medicine. I had practiced for 25 years in Florida before becoming an academic physician.

It is often the case in life that something unexpected, something that challenges our very existence, our mortality, our stability, occurs. In my life, that challenge came after a biopsy of my prostate, a biopsy that returned a diagnosis of prostate cancer: a diagnosis that turned my life upside-down. It was this challenge, and the management of this challenge, that has led me to this narrative. This event shaped me in unlooked-for ways and its consequences became "the winter of my discontent." And yet, this time was not totally devoid of pleasure and humor, although intermingled with pain and uncertainty as to my future. A similar tale could be, and undoubtedly is being told many times over, in households throughout the world.

I hope that perhaps, by telling my story, my readers will be better able to deal with a similar challenge in each of their lives, and perhaps maintain in some ways their sense of humor, pleasure, dignity, and, most of all, love for their dear ones. "Hot Flashes in a Cold World," then, is my memoir of this life-changing event and the events that followed.

Chapter Two
AFTER DIAGNOSIS

The day that six needle biopsies of my prostate gland showed cancer in three of the six, my life was irrevocably changed– in an instant. From that day forward I was no longer a healthy, practicing physician, but now also a patient with an uncertain future,and a husband with perhaps another type of uncertain future. It is this story that I feel needs to be told and, perhaps, for those of you facing a similar challenge, the telling of it will be meaningful, enlightening and, I hope, helpful. Perhaps my being a physician as well as a patient will offer an added dimension, a slightly different perspective from that of non-physician patients with cancer or other life-threatening illness.

The biopsies, performed by a urologist, were done through a small instrument called an ultrasound probe, which was inserted into my rectum. A biopsy needle was introduced and six separate biopsies made, sampling six different areas of the prostate gland. This procedure determined whether I had prostate cancer, how extensive the cancer was within the prostate gland and how malignant the cancer was. It might also tell if the malignancy had spread outside of the prostate capsule, meaning that the cancer was not localized or confined to the prostate gland. The biopsies did, indeed cause concern, as they found prostate cancer with a very high Gleason score of nine.

This score was very meaningful, as the higher the Gleason score, the more poorly differentiated the cancer cells which means they were more malignant and carried a poorer prognosis than prostate cancer with a low score. In addition, the fact that the cancer could be felt on digital rectal examination strongly suggested that the cancer was not confined to the prostate and was, therefore, considered "locally invasive." It is true that prostate cancer can often be treated successfully, but the above findings were most worrisome. If the cancer is palpable or can be felt on examination as mine was it is considered inoperable, that is, it cannot be cured by surgery, and therefore carries a worse prognosis. The treatment, if surgery is not considered curative, is radiation in some form, or medicine to reduce the testosterone level since testosterone is what drives the cancer. These medicines are anti-androgens.

On May 18, 1993, my PSA was 0.8. On June 4, 1996, my PSA was 1.6, and January 12, 1998, 20 months later, it was 3.1. The PSA, or prostate-specific antigen, is a protein produced by cells of the prostate gland. If this blood test is elevated it may indicate the presence of prostate cancer and is therefore called a biological marker, or a tumor marker. I was having some symptoms of prostatic outlet obstruction but assumed this was due to a benign enlargement of my prostate gland. The urologist who checked me did not seem too alarmed, and told me to check the PSA again in a few months, as a rise in the PSA level might indicate the presence of prostate cancer.

I should have paid more attention when my PSA went up. Either I didn't want to worry or didn't think of myself having cancer, so I waited about six months and the repeat PSA May 12, 1998, was 2.8, which gave me some reassurance, since it hadn't risen further in the six months. That was eight months ago. I shouldn't have felt so secure. I had watched Janet's sister wait for the results of every CA-125 (a marker for ovarian cancer), and I couldn't imagine I would start doing the same with my PSA. It's a strange feeling, how the results of one test could set your mood, but here it was, happening to me. I waited for my next PSA, which was done on February 3, 1999, eight months later,(and had it done at that time only because my wife's sister was dying and Janet asked if I had checked my PSA. This time it was 12.4! I was in shock, totally devastated and yet numb, not believing. I repeated it five days later and it came back 11.8 with an outside laboratory. Moreover, if prostate cancer is present, there is an additional test that distinguishes the total amount of prostate-specific antigen from the portion that is called *"free."* If the percentage of *"free"* PSA is less than 12 percent, there is a high probability that prostate cancer is present. When I saw my *"free"* PSA at less than 10 percent I knew I had prostate cancer.

I went to see a colleague and urologist at the Medical College of Georgia, and this time he felt a thickened area on the right side of my prostate, but he still felt it could be inflammation because the PSA went up so fast. He wanted me to take antibiotics for a few months, as prostatitis or inflammation of the prostate could give this rapid PSA change. I insisted on a biopsy, which he agreed to, but couldn't schedule for six weeks. Emotionally I couldn't wait and he knew it. The soonest he could arrange for a transrectal, ultra-sound- guided prostate biopsy was six weeks. He never made a move to get it done sooner. I almost felt he was only doing it to appease me, but I made the appointment.

When Janet, my wife, lover, friend and advocate, called me that night, she was furious: "There is no way you are waiting six weeks." And she was right. So I called Murray Freedman, my good friend, and two hours later I was in J.J. Carswell's office being examined. Carswell, a highly respected urologist in private practice, said too much of what the first urologist had said, and felt the same abnormality in my prostate, which was of concern to him. He arranged to do the biopsy in two days. And, as we had planned, one day after the biopsy, while I was seeing my own patients with my medical students, Janet, my wife, called Dr. Carswell, my urologist, to get the results. I was too nervous to call him myself.

I left so much to Janet, too much perhaps. It was after three in the afternoon and she hadn't called me and I knew she knew, so I called her. She just said, "come home," through her tears, and I knew I had cancer. I knew I had cancer without hearing it from her, knew it at some instinctive level. From that day forward, I was no longer a healthy, practicing physician and medical school professor but now also a patient with an uncertain future, and a husband with perhaps another type of uncertain future.

When I got home that day we just held each other and cried. I told her I didn't want to leave her, couldn't imagine being without her, couldn't believe I was dying. Our life together now seemed to have been so short, and could it really be near its end?

Never is there a good time for something like this, but we were waiting for the biopsy results while Janet was with her sister, Marcia, who was dying of ovarian cancer. We therefore would have to deal with Marcia's imminent demise and my cancer at the same time. It was as if Janet's sister, with ovarian cancer, was going to be replaced by Janet's husband, with prostate cancer.

I guess most of all I couldn't believe this was happening to me. I was at a wonderful place in my life. Janet and I were so content with our love, our home, our work. My job at the Medical College of Georgia was everything I wanted. I was taking care of patients, teaching medical students and residents how to do the same, and developing our medical school ethics curriculum. I felt appreciated and respected and, more than ever, I understood the need for teachers to be clinicians and humanitarians. That is what we were trained to be in my generation and, thank God, there were still some of us left. To us not every murmur was an "ejection murmur" and we didn't ask right away what the echo showed or what the ejection fraction was. And we were willing to let the patient tell us what was wrong. We not only listened but we heard, and heard with all our senses. So I liked what I was doing. And my love for Janet grew more intense and I needed her more, depended on her more every day.

Why the urologist at the Medical College of Georgia (MCG), where I was an associate professor of medicine, didn't appreciate our anxiety level and arrange to do the biopsy immediately is beyond me. I guess one would have to chalk it up to an insensitivity of the physician. So we turned to a private urologist in town. He agreed with the MCG urologist about it "possibly being inflammation," but did the biopsy within three days, realizing Janet's and my own need for confirmation.

Certainly, not waiting longer was appropriate. The three biopsies on the right side were positive for prostate cancer, with a Gleason score of 8 or 9. The pathologists had a difference of opinion about the biopsies from the left side, as to whether there was a low-grade cancer present or not. So I had a stage T2 b or c cancer, depending on whether there was bilateral involvement or not. The bone scan and CT scan were negative but there was little comfort to be drawn there, since gross metastases are seen in only a small percentage of cases. The staging conclusion was based on the high Gleason score and the fact that the cancer could be felt when my prostate was examined. These findings suggested that the cancer was "locally invasive."

Perhaps because Janet was 16 years younger than me, my physical wellbeing was terribly important to me. I had always been a competitive tennis player, from my high school days on. My college team at Oberlin was undefeated two years running and I played number two doubles and number three singles. I never stopped playing after that, including during my years in practice in Florida and after coming to Augusta. And I had been jogging for 30 years, literally every day, as well as tennis and work. My stamina was excellent. I always used to joke that as long as I could jog, play tennis, have functioning intact Betz cells and make love to my wife, not necessarily in that order, I would be OK.

I could not conceive of not being able to physically make love to Janet. I think not being impotent had been of vital importance to me throughout my adult life. So being faced with the need for neo-adjuvant therapy before and during radiation therapy was a tremendous blow to me. Hearing the words "chemical castration" was to me, the ultimate degradation. How could I go through with this? Janet, above all else, didn't want me to distance myself from her, to stop loving her.

We talked and held each other and cried and talked some more. And, two days after my biopsy, Janet and I left our Augusta home for a few days in Atlanta. I was attending an American Medical Association meeting on "Educating Physicians on End-of-Life Care." How ironic, I thought, for me to be at a meeting to help educate me on how to educate other physicians on how to deal with death and dying issues. I was now faced not only with teaching end-of-life care, but sometime, perhaps in the near future, receiving end-of-life care myself.

My son, Jeff, an orthopedic surgeon, arranged to come to Atlanta to be with us, bringing my 14-month-old granddaughter, Ally. What a mixture of sadness and joy, seeing them, and feeling the contrast between life beginning and life ending.

My wife wrote in her journal, "I cannot start at the beginning. The beginning is too sad and too difficult to find. Endings and beginnings are all tangled up together like a swami's basket of snakes. Many years ago there were beginnings that were happy, even glorious, and some endings—well, they were happy in their own way. They signified a turning point, a new direction that would make life sweeter once the difficulty that accompanies change had passed. Now changes are odious and unwelcome; now changes seem to mean profound sadness.

"I cannot think of a place to start that doesn't make me cry. I will not describe the end of my sister's struggle with cancer, nor the day I was told that my husband must begin his. There were only five days that separated those two events. And the beginning for Alan came even before the end for Marcia.

This family tragedy, for that is what it has been for all of us, started in 1993, just months after Alan and I had moved to Augusta. … What a wonderful opportunity for us both. We were immediately happy and thrilled with our decision. We felt life had never been better and, for us, it had always been so sweet.

And then everything changed. I cannot forget the Saturday morning Marcia and Billy called and asked that we both pick up the phone. I knew it must be bad news, but I did not even try to imagine what. It was "ovarian cancer." I was on the staircase and felt as though I had been punched hard in the stomach. I went down, sat and grasped myself at the waist. I was dazed and incredulous. I felt I knew the end of this story. Karen, my other sister and I spent hours on the phone trying to make sense of it. It would never make sense."

Chapter Three
BEGINNING TREATMENT

May 15, 1999

What a bizarre feeling the day I went down to Radiation Oncology at the New England Medical Center and had my first *conformal intensity-modulated radiotherapy*. (This is a form of radiotherapy or radiation to treat and hopefully destroy the prostate cancer cells.) I didn't know how to be a patient and not a doctor. To be reduced to this humble state, to be the cancer patient, was almost to be degraded, dehumanized, a person without an identity, without a persona. And yet, isn't that just what we ask our patients to be? I do believe every physician should have to be a patient as part of his medical training. I know now, what my father meant when, dying of heart disease and in the coronary care unit, and still practicing medicine, he turned to me and said, "At least I am dying with my stethoscope on."

My son Gary called that evening. He wanted to know whether I was getting chemotherapy. At first I said no, but then again I had received a four-month injection of leuprolide two months earlier after the biopsy. This is an anti-androgen, or, literally chemical castration. It has about the same effect as having your testicles surgically removed. I was also taking casodex, or bicalutamide, and the combination of the two was what is known as complete androgen blockade. That was hormonal therapy, since those medicines are anti-androgens. So I explained to him that perhaps I was getting a form of chemotherapy, albeit my treatments here were *conformal IMRT (intensity-modulated radiotherapy)*. This is a way of delivering more radiation just to the prostate rather than to the prostate and surrounding tissue such as the bladder and rectum.

No, it didn't mean my bone marrow would be temporarily severely affected, or that I would have severe nausea or acute ill feeling, or that I would lose my hair. No, I only had to put up with a lack of testosterone. So now I had hot flashes day and night. This was really something. The night's sleep was awful. Now I know what menopause and hot flashes are all about. I covered up and then awoke in a sweat, threw off the covers and got too cold with evaporation of sweat, covered up ... and so the night went. And not to be able to feel that testosterone surge was too dismal. But you know what? I didn't get to choose. This was what it took to have a shot at controlling this cancer and I wanted to have more time with Janet, so I did it. But if the price got too high, if all my dignity and function got hammered, if life was suffering, if Janet became a caretaker and me unable to have those things that make up my quality of life, then I would rethink my options. At this point, I could still work, my mind was clear; I could still jog, although it was getting to be more of a shuffle; I could still play tennis; and I could still hold my wife (my life), and sometimes even make love.

Speaking of a testosterone surge, for the first one or two weeks after getting leuprolide, the resulting testosterone surge was quite remarkable. For that time we were able to enjoy love-making, but what a mixed bag. It was such a mixture of loving feelings, sadness and closeness and gratification, fulfillment, despair, completion; and, on top of it, we wondered if this unexpected potency meant that the leuprolide wasn't working, that the cancer was growing unabated. What irony!

When I went out to jog the morning of my second day of XRT treatment, I couldn't help but laugh, imagining the Boston Globe headline: "68-year-old Physician and New England Medical Center Cancer Patient Seen Jogging Through the Boston Common While Receiving Radiation Therapy"! I did get some strange looks, come to think of it.

Then followed another uncomfortable night with hot flashes, sudden sweating and then coldness. Anyone who has ever had a radiology study using an intravenous iodinated dye such as an IVP (and many peri-menopausal women as well) will have some idea what these vasomotor episodes I was having were like. With both such radiation and menopause-related hot flashes a sudden build-up of heat goes all through your body. With the IVP the feeling begins in your head and overwhelms you with its forceful heat. There is an apprehension that goes with it also, but otherwise a very similar feeling.

I went out to run the following morning, if you could call it running. Sometimes it seemed more like a very slow trot. When I returned, Janet was still in bed. I wanted so much to make love to her and felt so deprived without testosterone. We were both doing the best we knew how, but it was not easy. As much closeness and love and sharing and trust and dependency as we had, there was still an element missing when we could not physically join. A part of our relationship was missing. We could talk about it and even joke about it, but it still hurt.

Later, I e-mailed Dan Rahn, then Acting Chief of the Section of General Internal Medicine, and Bill Strong, a fellow faculty member. They were—are—two of my very good friends and support team. Bill said he was keeping the prayers going and Sts. Francis and Jude were two of his heroes who did good work. My son Marc said that he and Louise were doing the same.

Dan was a wonderful support and sounding-board throughout my illness. He never failed to spend some time every day talking to me. He is remarkably perceptive and sensitive. He also has a deep, abiding religious faith, as does Janet. I had not yet adopted their same attitude of resignation, but hearing of it helped. Janet is certain we will never be apart, that I will always be with her, and after we both died we will be together forever.

Dan told me that this cancer would test my spirit, and every day I had found this to be so true. But it was so important to have a support system, to have people to talk to, people who love you, and respect you, and care about you, as you about them. And, to actively be doing something. I think being depressed is mostly about feeling helpless and angry. If you are actively doing something you won't feel so helpless and, if you have loved ones to share all your feelings with, perhaps you won't feel as angry.

My son Jeff called that night and told me that his wife Sharon's ultrasound of her fetus (she was due that October and she was in her late thirties) showed a choroid plexus cyst, possibly indicating spina bifida or other congenital anomalies. They were now waiting for the results of the amniocentesis, so were obviously anxious. They wouldn't know for seven to 10 days. Sharon hadn't told me when I spoke to her two nights earlier, because she didn't think I needed anything else to worry about. This was understandable, but my having cancer was hardly an insulation against all else that went on in my life. It was a great concern, of course, but so were many other things. I was not so totally absorbed with my cancer that all else was excluded—I hoped that would never be.

Thursday, I awakened after sleeping much longer than I usually do. I planned to have an apple for breakfast. The idea was to eat fruits and vegetables while I still could, because by the following week there would more than likely be symptoms of proctitis/colitis (inflammation of the rectum and large intestine), as well as bladder and prostate inflammation from the radiation. At that time I would need to follow a low-residue diet, so fruits and vegetables would have to be restricted.

That morning I had zero appetite and seemed a little sluggish. This was an interesting paradox. Was I feeling this way because I was out of my routine, or because of the radiation, or what? And I worried about Janet not eating just because I was not, and feeling she had to keep me company. She didn't need to not eat. I usually took care of preparing her meals as much as I could, and I might not be able to do so for a while. Janet says nobody starves who has food available—maybe so, but I think she has an anorectic outlook. Anyway I went down for my fourth treatment that morning.

I was such a creature of habit. I needed my routine and I needed to be busy with a full day. At home, I usually started my day at 5:30 a.m. with a 45-minute jog or similar time on my Nordic, then worked all day, met Janet for lunch two or three times a week, then played tennis two or three evenings a week, and fixed dinner at least three times a week or more before I did some reading, and—at least before I became an iatrogenic eunuch, with a little bit of luck made love to my soulmate. So this existence was hard to put up with and I didn't know whether I felt off physically, or emotionally, or both.

Another interesting feature of being in this medical center was to be in a cancer unit residence where all the other occupants were cancer patients, and to go, as they all did, with their families, to the radiation oncology treatment unit where we received our treatment. I tell you, it didn't leave any doubt in your mind that you had cancer. Dan Rahn used to tell me that getting through this would take a lot of spirit and he was so right. It was literally one "insult" after another. It was almost as if you got no chance to deal with one affront before another hit you. And you had no help from the staff. There was no tender, loving care, nobody asking you what you were thinking or feeling. Thank God for Janet. Did every patient going through this assault have a Janet? I didn't think so.

Have you read Solzhenitsyn's "Cancer Ward?" This is a very depressing business.

We decided to drive up to our home in Friendship, Maine, following a Friday morning treatment. It would be good to be in our own home with our own things, our own "rules," our own schedule, our own routine. I think it might be easier if one went through this in one's home, with one's usual surroundings, rather than far away in foreign surroundings.

I was beginning to feel a physical discomfort in my rectum, like a feeling of unrest in my bowels, like an impending need to evacuate, and in a hurry; and yet, not that bad yet, but a harbinger of things to come. You see, each development was a new assault, a new indignity, another taking away, of and from. Now I had zero appetite, no desire for food whatsoever. In fact, thinking of eating actually aggravated that feeling in my bowels. First, my sexual desire was taken away. It went with my testosterone. Then, my desire for food was gone. That still left me with jogging, tennis and a functioning cerebral cortex. So I could complain—what, up to 40 percent?

Struggling to adjust to this new time in my life also made me remember what my father said to me when he was forced to semi-retire and spend a few winter months in Florida in the town where I practiced medicine.

I visited him at lunchtime as he sat at poolside playing cards with his men friends, all retired or in Florida for the winter. "Everything is called living," he said. That is what he felt not being at work caring for his patients. I now know how he felt.

The quintessential old-time physician: When I think of my father I think of him as just that. He was an old-time clinician, the "family doc" who delivered babies, literally on the kitchen table if need be, made house calls, held Sunday "rounds" for the relatives, answered the phone while having dinner—which usually lasted 15 minutes, from 6 to 6:15 p.m.—and then went down to the office until 8 p.m. In those days there was no phone answering system with 10 different choices. No, in those days when you wanted to talk to your doctor you got to talk to your doctor. No one ran interference for him and no one kept his patients from talking to him. (Well, come to think of it, my mother did, at least at dinnertime and sometimes on weekends. She became quite good at telling patients to take a couple of aspirin, and knowing when they really needed to talk to "Doctor Dave.") He was always quick to say "you'll live" when we approached him, my brother Marty and I, with this ache or that ache, and yet he had that innate ability to know what was serious and what wasn't. Nothing seemed to ruffle his feathers.

In many ways Cliff Turner, my attending at the 35th Street Clinic in downtown Cleveland, Ohio, when I was a third-year medical student, reminded me of my Dad. When we were presenting a sick baby to Cliff he would come into the examining room, walk around the table upon which the baby was being examined, looking at the baby but not touching, and finally say, "That's a real sick baby." He was invariably right.

My father opened his office on Rochambeau Avenue in the Bronx in 1926. You could see P.S. 80 from the office window on the first floor. The office was part of the apartment we lived in, although I was not yet born, nor was my brother, Marty. But when we did begin elementary school it was P.S. 80 we went to. Rochambeau Avenue and Mosholu Parkway, where we moved to next, were somewhere between Jerome Avenue, the Grand Concourse and 205th Street. This part of the Bronx was inhabited mostly by Jews and Italians, a smattering of Irish, and not much else. If you walked up to 205th Street, you could get your prescriptions filled at Dobris' Drug Store by Mr. Dobris himself; or get an egg cream soda at Levy's corner candy store. A few stores down was Crimi's barber shop, with haircuts by Mr. Crimi or his second barber in one of the two or three chairs that made up the shop. Another few stores down was the delicatessen where the kosher hot dogs were grilling on a gas grill right inside the big front plate-glass window. Next to the hot dogs were barrels of new and more seasoned pickles, and big containers of fresh sauerkraut. Some years later I learned to know this "deli" quite well, since I walked by it every afternoon, five days a week, on my way to Hebrew School at the Mosholu Jewish Center, which was our synagogue or "schul." By that time we had moved around the corner to Mosholu Parkway, which was a step up, I guess, because it fronted a park with trees and grass and across the park was the Grand Concourse. In those days, you could get pony rides, join the other kids in winter to sled down the small slope of the park, and sit around the big boulder in the park, build a small fire to keep warm and even roast "spuds— that is, until my Dad would call the police because he was afraid we would burn ourselves.

Getting back to Rochambeau Avenue and Doctor Dave, well, talk about serendipity. When my Dad opened his office as a general practitioner in 1926, one of the first patients to come to his office was a woman with large varicose veins on her legs who wanted them removed or at least shrunk if possible. My Dad had never treated anyone with varicose veins other than to refer them to a surgeon for vein stripping or vein ligation, both of which were surgical procedures. However, he had heard of a new medicine, a sclerosing agent called sodium morrhuate, that, when injected into the varicose vein, caused the vein to sclerose and lose its blood flow, thereby contracting and sometimes even disappearing. Since he had never done this before, he asked the patient if she would return in one week, at which time he would have the necessary medicine. He then went to the medical library and read how the procedure was done, and obtained the medicine. In his reading, it was emphasized that the sodium morrhuate was extremely caustic and could damage the skin and tissue around the vein if any of it was allowed to leak out during the injection. In fact, in the protocol, it stated that if the physician saw any swelling of the tissue or skin where the needle was placed as the medicine was injected, the physician should immediately withdraw the needle and try again at another time. Being scrupulously honest, he explained all of this to the patient, and then proceeded to prep the area and begin the treatment. No sooner had he started to inject when a small swelling developed and he immediately withdrew the needle, apologized to the patient and told her he had not injected any medicine into the vein, and would not charge her for the visit since he had accomplished nothing, but was willing to try again another time.

One week later, the woman whose varicose vein he was unable to inject, called to thank him for his excellent treatment as the vein had shrunk and had virtually disappeared, and she wanted to return to pay him for his services. He tried to explain to her that he had done nothing, but she believed he was just being modest. Of course, it's possible that a small amount of the drug had caused a reaction around the vein, leading to its collapse and unexpected shrinkage. In any case, soon thereafter, another woman called, wanting her varicose veins treated, and then another, and, within a few months he had an established practice largely treating varicose veins. In point of fact, he became the varicose vein specialist of Rochambeau Avenue and the South Bronx.

Chapter Four

I CAN BREATHE AGAIN

Friday, May 21, 1999 found us finally back in Friendship. What a blessing. I had not realized how oppressive it was to go from a cancer residence facility at the Tufts-New England Medical Center, living with all the other cancer patients, to the Radiation Oncology Unit, receiving treatment with those same cancer patients. Now, it felt like I could breathe again for the first time in two weeks. I actually felt better that day, although with no appetite, and with that feeling of my bottom being on the verge of falling out. My energy level was good and I was not as teary and as up-and-down with my emotions, so a lot of my discomfort must have been, and was, emotional.

Two nights earlier, Tom DePetrillo, my radiation oncologist, had given us his two tickets to the Boston Red Sox/Yankees baseball game at Fenway Park. This was quite an honor, as Boston fans are so very rabid. Tom, chief of radiation oncology at Tufts New England

Medical Center, was giving a lecture in California and had to miss the game and was good enough to offer the tickets to us. With the Red Sox and Yankees battling for first place, this was something. We sat in his box right behind the first base dugout and it was wonderfully exciting. The next night we went to the Boston Ballet's performance of "Dracula," which was very good and helped our mood a bit. But nothing was like getting away from Boston and being in my own house in the woods, looking out to the sea.

I do believe, in some ways, doctors who are patients are treated differently, and not necessarily to their advantage. They are neither fish nor fowl and I think the staff doesn't exactly know how to treat them.

My wife wrote, "For Alan, it is the worst possible scenario to be in a hospital and be a patient, not a doctor. For me, it feels like an invasion of our privacy somehow. I feel we are somehow exposed by sharing waiting rooms with people we don't know, and nurses who call him 'Mr. Roberts.' The title 'Dr.' never seemed to be important before, but now, to call him 'Mr.' somehow robs him of a very essential part of himself. He is somehow reduced to something less than he was before this diagnosis."

Janet and I had been talking about whether it would be a good idea for the residents of Neely House—all of them undergoing some form of cancer treatment— and their families, to have some roundtable discussions about what they were going through, their feelings, etc. Sometimes talking about one's illness with others and hearing what they are going through is a form of therapy. There is a certain comfort for many patients when they can discuss their anxiety, their emotions and what they are going through with others—sort of group therapy. What is more, I thought that it might prove of value to have someone with my background as a physician and educator, and then cancer patient, to facilitate such a discussion.

I was uncertain I would want to do it, but Janet's response was that, for her, she wouldn't want it. One of our first nights there, she had written in her journal, "It is 10 p.m. and I sit in this room, watching Alan sleep and working a 1,000-piece puzzle. Every 20 minutes, I go to the laundry room to swap from washer to dryer, to fold, etc. In these quiet halls I occasionally cross paths with other residents. Mostly, I believe I see family members and caretakers. Sometimes, I see a bald young man or two. They are much younger than we and have lots more life to live. I keep feeling like it is so very sad that they are here enduring this ordeal. I don't feel at all related. I don't feel as though we are facing what they might be facing. They are families with cancer. They are facing the loss of a son, a brother, and maybe a husband. I can't identify at all. While I have felt little optimism since Alan's diagnosis, since we have moved into the Neely House I feel a sense of distance from this disease, as though all these other residents are in a battle for their lives but we are just spending time here. I feel guilty taking the space from someone who perhaps really needs it. I don't think I am fooling myself, yet I am able to completely distance myself from our situation."

Janet felt that, giving voice to the issues related to why we were here would only make things more real, and somehow more tangible. If left unsaid, it would sort of stay at a distance, be less distinct, less intrusive.

Somehow, for her, talking about it gave it shape and form and brought it closer. And yet she and I talked about it a lot—but just the two of us, alone. How interesting life is. Sometimes I wish Janet and I weren't so close and didn't love so intensely, but then I don't think that would have helped us get through this time in our lives, with its inevitable outcome, with any greater ease. And I cannot imagine living without feeling what I have been allowed to feel. What a gift and blessing—yes, it makes everything more intense, the good and the bad, but I think better to feel this way than not at all.

The next morning, I awakened in my home in the Maine woods. It was so good to feel alive. We'd stopped for lunch the day before on the way to Friendship, at a little roadside restaurant near Wiscasset. It was called the Sea Basket and was right across the street from Al's Discount Store on Route 1. The variety of items Al carried with a low price tag and great utilitarianism was amazing. After a little shopping, our lunch was wonderful. Janet had a lobster roll and I had a bowl of fish chowder that was piping hot and filled with chunks of light, fresh haddock and new potatoes. If you have never had Maine new potatoes you are missing a special experience. What a treat. And our meal at home the night before had consisted of fresh broccoli, baked new potatoes with chives and butter, and a piece of wonderfully fresh salmon poached in white wine and lemon juice with dill, on my electric barbeque grill. There is really nothing like fresh fish from cold North Atlantic waters. I hadn't realized how deprived I was, staying in Boston with a toaster oven and microwave to cook on.

Of course, that was only a small part of what I was feeling. Staying at the hospital was so oppressive and I didn't fully appreciate that until I got away from there. Looking back on it, I realize that most of what I was feeling was depression. I don't know if you remember the comedian Dick Shawn, but he had a routine when stereo music was being popularized in which he talked about the ultimate stereo experience, which was to build a house out of a huge speaker and to live inside it. Well, that is exactly what it felt like living in the Neely House in the medical center. It was like living inside a cancer— as if that is all there was. I was engulfed, enshrouded in cancer and my lost energy was all stress-induced.

How did I know? Well, for one thing, when I got out of bed that weekend, the world didn't seem at all oppressive. I saw and felt the beauty of the pristine Maine woods. I dressed and jogged for 53 minutes without any strain, including the two hills between my house and the village. When I returned home I dug clams for lunch—soft-shell clams, good for steaming. Digging clams is a chore—it is done with a six-prong pitchfork cut off to have only a 12-to-14 inch handle and bent at 90 degrees or more. At low tide you look for holes in the muck and lift pieces of muck with the clamming rake, or clamming fork as it is properly called. Usually, you can see clams sticking in the underside of the muck. Or sometimes they shoot a stream of water, which is not only interesting but helps identify their location. After an hour or so of this, it often isn't easy to straighten up, but the effort is well worth it.

I then waxed about half of our Explorer, drove into Rockland to antique shop and finally home to eat lunch at 2 p.m. After such a day I had no doubt about my energy level, but also marveled at how badly I had felt one day earlier in Boston. I don't think we give enough attention to the spirit of our patients. My radiation oncologist had warned me of some loss of energy with my treatments and I was willing to accept this as due to the treatments, when in reality it was due to my emotional state. I didn't doubt I would suffer some loss of energy but one's spirit is of vital importance. I think managed care would cost our healthcare delivery system more in the long run than a single-payer system, or perhaps even fee-for-service, if it didn't allow enough time for physician-patient encounters and an awareness of the need for enough time for proper counseling. Without such time, the cost of additional treatment would be far greater. Of course, as an old-time clinician, I can say with complete confidence that seeing 20 to 40 patients a day to meet managed-care guidelines can never allow for medical care as it needs to be practiced.

I rounded out the day by making dinner, followed by a game of Boggle. Then I hoped to maybe get lucky and find my body parts responsive. I made crab cakes, with fresh crabmeat and little else, baked sweet potatoes with brown sugar and butter, and boiled beets with butter. (When I say butter, you know I mean a butter substitute).

Well, I didn't get lucky that night or the following morning, although I did feel a little responsiveness and that was good. Amazing how we can settle for less; even a crumb is better than none! Cancer and the necessary involvement of the cancer doctors (or oncologists) doing the treating makes for an oppressive, omnipresent, all-encompassing force. When you are in its thrall, nothing else can compete.

I have long wondered why sexual ability and potency mean so much to me. It is more than part of expressing my love and closeness to Janet. I think it has something to do with my feelings of self-esteem, of being a man, and perhaps even part of my need to achieve. I have never done anything halfway, sexual functioning included.

I awakened Sunday morning feeling blessed and very lucky, in spite of my cancer. The light shining in through our skylight loft windows above our bed, the trees swaying in the breeze, the sunlight glinting off the water, the quiet of the Maine woods. So quiet you could hear the quiet, it seemed. All of this, with Janet next to me, made me feel blessed. I did want to thank God for having given me all this. However long I had to live—and, believe me, I was not ready to leave all of this—but, however long, I counted it as a blessing. I hoped my treatments would give me a lot of years. I am naturally not very optimistic and did not envision a long period of relapse-free survival, especially with a Gleason score of 8 or 9. But, whatever, right that moment, I counted my blessings.

We planned to walk four or five miles on Martin's Point, which juts out into Muscongus Bay on the other side of Friendship Harbor. Later, we would ride into Waldoboro where the county trash disposal site is located 10 miles or so from Friendship, pick up some scallions for my home-made potato soup that we would have for dinner that night, and enjoy clearing some fallen trees and such around our house. I wanted to get my inflatable, a small Zodiac, ready to put into the water.

I used it to get us out to my boat, which was moored just beyond the tidal water in back of our cottage. Our lobsterman/house-watcher had been good enough to rig a mooring with a 75-pound mushroom anchor and a red ball float within view of my back windows. What a lovely site. I had a small boat that was quite sufficient for my purposes but would wait until the following weekend to put it on the mooring. The following day, we had to return to New England Medical Center for my sixth XRT, and I intended to savor all of that day.

The next morning, we awoke with the sound of rain on the roof and the wind through the trees. The water was rough enough to form small whitecaps with the tide half in. Well, guess what? I actually made love to Janet. I cannot describe to you how wonderful it was to be able to be physically intimate with my wife. I do not know why it was so important—it just was. Without that intimacy, it felt as if something was missing. I thanked God for that gift today. After some time we talked of our mortality, Janet and I. It was so hard for me to think of leaving Janet and the life I loved so much, and to think of being in the process of dying. But Janet said, in response, "We're all dying, Al." I guess that was so, and it put a different slant on where I was and what I was feeling.

In beginning this tale, thoughts of my childhood arose, thoughts that had been hidden, it seemed, in the recesses of my subconscious for so many years, and now suddenly began to surface; thoughts I feel compelled to briefly relate, perhaps because, over the ensuing years, there seems so very little of my childhood that has captured my thoughts, so little that I have relived, or, in many cases, barely remembered. Sadly, most of what I recall was not so pleasant, and that perhaps accounts for its latency for so long. There is, however, in these memories, a person who, in some ways, I think, kept me feeling something other than anger, unhappiness, and resentment. That person was Essie, our live-in housekeeper and, in the truest sense of the words, my nanny. Thinking of Essie, even so many years later, fills me with the feelings of a warm, enfolded, emotional embrace. Yes, there are other good memories, to be sure, but thinking of Essie is so much more than a pleasant memory. For me, having Essie was having a mother, comforter, friend. She represented security, and most important, unconditional love. And at the same time, she was someone in need of all that herself.

I do not know why my childhood seems, looking back, so difficult, so cold and uncomforting, so bleak in many ways. Perhaps because that's really how it was. At first glance, an objective observer might have seen it as idyllic. My father was a successful physician in the practice of family medicine, a "general practitioner" as he was known then, residing in a comfortable middle class neighborhood in the Bronx. I was born in 1930, so you get the idea of the times.

My mother was emotionally very fragile, sustaining several serious depressions. My father treated her, in many ways, as a child, which must have suited him well, but may not have served her so. After he died, in fact, she showed remarkable ability to live independently and care for herself. Early on, he not only practiced but did the food shopping, took care of all the family finances, made the major decisions; and my mother shopped, going almost every day on the subway, to and from home, to Madison Avenue and Fifth Avenue. If she became depressed, my father's treatment consisted of letting her redecorate the apartment, or buy another fur coat, or sending her to Florida for a month during the winter. And if all else failed, there were electroshock treatments with a psychiatrist and family friend, Bill Karliner.

My parents loved me, I know, but my mother was unable to be comfortable with any outward expression of love. She just wasn't comfortable enough with herself, and was filled with insecurity and self-doubt. I do not remember her ever saying, "I love you." And yet, I knew she did. My father, on the other hand, just didn't know how to express his love, other than by providing us with all the amenities, making sure I had an algebra tutor when I needed one, and such. I grew up angry … angry that he could give so freely to his patients and friends and extended family but seemingly not to me, and not to my brother, Marty. I am certain he never for a moment thought he was depriving us of anything. What a sad thing.

I wonder how many other children of doctors felt so deprived. To everyone else he was a God, but I felt cheated, and angry. As a child, it was very difficult living with a God and trying to live up to his expectations. So my childhood was full of "sick headaches," as Essie called them, and nightmares that kept me crawling into my older brother's bed for comfort. But the real comfort came from Essie. With Essie, there was security and love and caring. There was a cloth soaked in vinegar for my headaches, a book full of numbers to look up and to bet a few pennies on my dreams, though I doubt, even with the proper number, that she ever collected those few cents—this, and so much more. (For those readers who are wondering how one can bet on a dream, in those days, and in Harlem, there were "dream books" and the subjects of dreams were assigned a certain number. And if you bet on the winning number you won a bet and collected some money. This is what Essie did with my dreams.)

On our way back from Maine, Janet and I talked about our first marriages and why they didn't work for either of us. For one thing I don't think I was capable of loving anyone at the time, no matter who or what. Janet thought that I could not have had a good, loving relationship without good, loving sexual intimacy and a woman who helped me feel good about myself.

The more I thought about it, I didn't think any loving relationship was possible until I dealt with my anger. This took years and much therapy, and finally a therapist who was able to help me feel how angry I was with my father. He was the all-giving, dedicated physician who had something to give to all his patients but so little to his family. Besides, everyone thought Dave was God. It wasn't easy living with God. How could I live up to his expectations? How could I be good enough?

And then he had to die before I could tell him how much I loved him and before he could tell me what I so needed to hear. He never did so in life and I was doubly angry that he died with two thoughts expressed to me at his deathbed in the coronary care unit. One I mentioned previously, about dying with his stethoscope on—just what I wanted to hear—not "I love you, or I will miss you, or you are a wonderful physician, too." And then he had to add, "Take care of your mother—you will have your hands full."

What a wonderful farewell. So it took me years with a skilled therapist to finally allow myself to let that anger out and to finally feel my love for my father. After that it became possible to love—something not possible before with my first wife or anyone else.

Chapter Five

LIFE IS A BATTLE

Back in Boston, and treatment number 12 was over. Up to this point, I had had few problems with the side effects of XRT. Perhaps there had been a slight feeling of increased urinary urgency, and a feeling of something going on in my bowels like I could evacuate at any time. My energy level had remained good, thanks to the gift of a weekend in Maine and my good physical conditioning to begin with.

But my thoughts were rather morbid that week. Wednesday had been a most difficult day and I was not certain I knew why. First of all, I had had three different dreams, all rather strange, and one of the three I hadn't retained. I didn't want to go into them. In addition, I seemed to have been in a sweat all night long and my mouth had felt thick and dry. I thought my breath must have reflected my discomfort. I had risen feeling tired but having to defecate, and again feeling a mixture of constipation and rectal irritation. Then back to bed. I was feeling very down and only wanted Janet to be close to me. In spite of all, I had found myself partially aroused and had been able to sustain a sort of erection, barely enough to achieve penetration. My feelings had been mixed—pleasure at being able to be that close to Janet and emotional pain at my feeble ability to make love to my wife. My thoughts had been all over the place and I couldn't help wondering whether it would be more painful to be without Janet at all at a time like this or whether it was more painful being an incomplete husband with cancer and no testosterone. And what would be best for Janet? There was something about not having testosterone that was so deadly. It took all my spirit to continue. Perhaps life should have ended before all of this happened, quickly and unexpectedly.

There is a story about a little boy sitting on the sidewalk crying, and an old man asks him why he is crying. The little boy responds by saying he is crying because he can't do what the big boys do. So the old man sits down and cries too. I feel like that old man.

Even after treatment number 12, I was not having a great deal of difficulty physically, but I did seem to be more tired and less energetic. The bowel and bladder symptoms were manageable. Mostly, I was feeling sad and I suppose depressed, and yet it was not constant.

Life is a battle. I have always considered myself a fighter. Winning, in everything I do, has always been vital to me. Because of this inner need I have attempted to maintain my proficiency in areas of skill and expertise in fields that I have felt were important to me. That has held true in my practice of medicine as well as in my physical wellbeing, and in the practice of those physical skills I have elected to pursue and in which I seemed to have some native talent.

While in high school (Hopkins Grammar School in New Haven, Conn.—the third oldest preparatory private school in the United States), I was able to graduate magna cum laude, third highest in the class. I was able to obtain admission to Yale University and Oberlin College. I chose Oberlin. My brother was in his third year at Yale, my cousin Marvin in his second year, my father had graduated from Yale Medical School and was born in New Haven, with most of his family still there although we lived in New York City. I just needed some fresh air, had to get away from the traditional pathway and chose a small liberal arts school in the Midwest with excellent credentials and an excellent record for getting students into graduate programs.

Well, while at Hopkins I played trumpet in the school orchestra, was captain of the tennis team and played number one, and was a starting guard on our basketball team. So you see, achieving was something I did not take lightly. I felt the same way about my practice of medicine and could not have been satisfied with less than my best, which meant being compulsively honest and meticulous; being in tight control of my patients, which was much easier then than it is now; and continuing to educate myself faithfully. That allowed me to maintain and increase my skills and knowledge base, which led me to certify in internal medicine, then re-certify—even though at the time I was not required to do so. I went on to earn Fellowship in the American College of Physicians, and finally to certify for Added

Qualifications in Geriatric Medicine the first year the certifying examination was given (1988), when I could be grandfathered in; that is, receive certification in geriatric medicine on the basis of passing the examination and being already certified in Internal Medicine and without having taken an approved residency in geriatric medicine as it had not been available when I trained.

My need to win kept me physically fit and competitive so that I could continue to play challenging, winning tennis—and do so even to this day, winning against much younger opponents and, in general, outlasting them if nothing else. It has allowed me to continue jogging virtually every day. Life is a constant battle. It takes meeting more and more obstacles, some through a natural process of aging and its deleterious effect, and some unexpected, such as tennis elbow and such. It is not only a battle but a whittling-away process. With age, everything becomes more of an effort and requires more energy and fortitude and willpower but, no matter what you do, it is a downhill course, inexorable, never-ending—except with death.

I didn't want to be so whittled away that I existed without the ability to do what I most love to do. I accepted my deteriorating game of tennis, my reduced jogging speed, the increased energy required to do it. I understood radiation treatments had a consequence but to me it was just another added burden, another call for additional reserves—but not an easy submission. I had to continue in what I needed to do to feel my self-worth. What I could not do I would try to abide by, but it was extremely difficult, and I particularly struggled with this impotence, with this loss of testosterone. But I would not give up. I hoped my anti-androgen treatments could be discontinued after the three to four months. I wanted that desperately. That part of my being seemed so important to me. Nothing in my relationship with Janet could fill that particular void.

Cancer is all-encompassing. It is a constant effort to keep it from being overwhelming. It would have been so easy to give in to it, but also so deadly—just as giving up my exercise and my work and my loving relationship with Janet would have been. Nobody said it would be easy, and I had told my patients countless times that getting old was not for sissies. Now, I counseled myself accordingly.

Friday was not a good day. I was still tearful and sad, although there was nothing specific. I guess I was depressed and yet, not exactly. My concentration and interest was off a bit but I was still getting some work done, although admittedly not as much as I should have been. I jogged in the morning for 40 minutes, had my 14th treatment and met with Tom DePetrillo for a few minutes.

If you haven't read William M. Landau's book "Clinical Neuromythology and other Arguments and Essays, Pertinent and Impertinent" (Futura Publishing Company Inc., Armonk, New York, 1998), I recommend it highly. The author assails the lack of clarity in medical writing and bemoans the fact that most house staff don't know the difference between a transitive and intransitive verb. He argues for a return to simple factual description, so that, for instance, we can describe how a patient walks slowly rather than saying that he demonstrates bradykinesia. I might add to this the fact that we, as physicians, too often talk in euphemisms and try to avoid presenting the blunt facts, if unfavorable, and instead use vague innuendo and meaningless phrases.

For example, Tom, my radiation oncologist, wanted me to have a CT scan the following Tuesday. A previous CT scan with contrast had revealed a small density outside, but near, the prostate. He wasn't sure this meant anything and Jim Rawson at MCG, when he initially read the scan, was not convinced that it represented metastatic disease. So when I had questioned Tom about the comparison with the second CT scan I had without contrast, before beginning radiation and after the stainless steel seeds were placed in my prostate, he had said something like, "There's just a little 'ditzel' there now." Well, what did that mean? Originally, if it had disappeared with treatment, it had probably represented a metastasis. Now he was saying it could be a lymph node. Then he said, "Whatever, the high Gray radiation will take care of it."

Okay, granted the answer was not clear. The scans were imperfect and we can only sometimes make an educated guess. Well, why not just say so? At this point I didn't know whether I had locally invasive cancer or just localized within the prostate, or metastatic. I would have liked to know because treatment might depend upon the conclusion. Whatever, I would hope the radiation would control the cancer. I was prepared for another three months of anti-androgen treatment but I could accept it only with the greatest reluctance. I truly could not come to terms with being unable to physically make love to my wife—at least, not without great difficulty.

I felt as if I were a burden to Janet and that was not a good feeling.

We need to make every effort as physicians to remove euphemisms and jargon and lack of candor from our conversations with patients. In some ways this is strange for me to say, as I have always been paternalistic and wanting to be in complete control of my patients. I still feel there are times when complete candor is more harmful than "fudging" here and there, but overall I think leveling with the patient, but as kindly and optimistically as possible, will be in the patient's best interest.

I must tell you about my Uncle Irving and Aunt Edie. They were my patients in Florida years ago when relatives came to live near their "nephew the doctor," who would take care of them. This was at a time when being physician to family was rather commonplace. By the way, I remember "Sunday rounds" as a child in New Haven, Conn. We lived in New York City, where my father practiced medicine. My father's mother, sister Ruth and her family, brother Irving and his family and sister Esther and her family lived in New Haven. We drove there almost every Sunday, and there my father had Sunday office hours—for the family!)

Back to Edie and Irving. One year, Irving came in for his annual checkup and his blood count had dropped, with the hematocrit down from 42 to 35 percent. A fecal occult blood test was positive. This reminds me of something an internist in Cleveland, Ohio, told me when he was interviewing me as a potential associate, as I was completing my residency. He said a good internist should do a thorough history and physical, a fecal occult blood test, a blood count and a urinalysis and he would miss very little. I believe that is largely true in spite of enormous technological advances since, and I still apply these principles in my patient care today.

Getting back to Uncle Irving; when I had the above results I ordered a barium enema X-Ray, which revealed a lesion in the hepatic flexure. He was scheduled for surgery, but I told the surgeon I didn't want him told he had cancer if that was the case. Rather, I asked him to tell Irving he had a polyp and it was completely removed. The cancer, which it was, was confined, had not invaded the adventitia or beyond, the liver was clean and so Irving was told he had a benign polyp. Several years later, his wife, my Aunt Edie, developed abdominal pain while in New York and was operated on by the same surgeon at Mt. Sinai Hospital who found a small bowel cancer, also confined and resectable. After discussion with me, he told her she had an intestinal abscess that was cured. We did tell Irv that Edie had small bowel cancer, and we told Edie that Irv had colon cancer, but neither of them ever knew they themselves had cancer. Irving died of Alzheimer's disease many years later in his eighties, and Edie died of small cell lung cancer many years later, also in her eighties.

Anyway, I still would have to await my next CT scan the following Tuesday, and hope for a good outcome.

Saturday was a beautiful day. The sun came up around 5 a.m., the air was dry and I had a great deal of energy. I was convinced any energy lack I had generally was emotional. I knew part of my problem was feeling inadequate, and most of that was from chemical castration, and not being at my desk and seeing patients.

I did so much better in Maine, it was unreal. During an earlier visit just before I began radiation treatment,

Janet had written, "When we crossed the state line from New Hampshire into Maine, I wanted to slam the door behind us, to resolve to stay here in our house in the woods where tragedy and pain cannot reach us. I don't want to leave this nest, this place that has been a serene, simple solace for the past 12 years. We built this house as an escape and now I am ready to shut the doors and leave the world outside for good."

You know, when we were driving up to Maine on Friday and I was feeling so low and we stopped to change drivers, Janet asked me to put my seat belt on. We always wore our seat belts. At that moment, the only thought I had was, "Why?" What difference did it make? I didn't say anything and I did put my seat belt on but that is how low I felt. And yet, I wanted to live, and for a long time. I didn't want to die. There was much yet to be done and I wanted to be with Janet, now, for a long time, and forever.

That weekend was absolutely glorious. My energy level was as good as ever and we landscaped the front of our house, took a five-mile walk, did a little fishing—although it was very windy out in the open water. I got my 2 H.P. Johnson running on my Zodiac to get out to my boat moored in deep water. It took a little "dry gas" but it ran like a charm, belying its 24 years.

We are situated on tidal water on the Meduncook River, which is an inlet of Muscongus Bay. Tides usually are about 12 feet in Maine, which means we have no navigable water at low tide in back of our house. That is where I harvest mussels and dig my soft-shell clams, ideal for steaming and I love them. So we did a lot of chores and had a wonderful time.

Chapter Six
SIDE EFFECTS

Week Number 4 of my treatment began with treatment Number 15. We got back to Boston well in time for my 3:00 P.M. appointment and met with Dr. McGrath to arrange for my CT scan on Wednesday, apparently for the evaluation of prostate volume for further treatments. Then to Government Center, to our P.O. Box to pick up our mail, and then a walk to Newbury Street through the Common. It was remarkably hot for this time of year at 95 degrees, and extremely humid. Although dressed for the heat I really felt fatigued and weak and uncomfortable. I stopped once to sit and drink a bottle of water, and was amazed at how much I was sweating. What a pleasure to get back to the Neely House, lie down and doze off before taking a shower. My spirits were better afterwards and I wanted to get down to the various tasks I planned to do.

The plan was to continue with radiation and the last three weeks would be conformal intensity-modulated radiotherapy. My side effects were tolerable but certainly present. Forgive me for boring you with all the details related to radiation treatment, but the GI side effects were most bothersome in that there was a constant abdominal malaise with episodic bowel spasms, total loss of appetite and a lot of noisy rumbling of the abdomen after eating, with an urge to defecate. Interestingly enough, local steroid usage such as proctofoam-HC helped with all of the symptoms, but the most comfortable solution was not to eat at all. Even liquids were bothersome. There was also a heaviness in my prostate, particularly noticeable when voiding—almost painful. In spite of it all, my energy level was still pretty good, although not normal. I jogged that morning for 42 minutes through the Boston Common, slowly but without having to stop, so I couldn't complain. I could have put up with it all a lot better, I think, if I hadn't been impotent. I was looking ahead to another 3 1/2 months of antiandrogens and impotency. I would be facing a great deal of difficulty emotionally and physically if the antiandrogens needed to be continued longer. How much must we give up to stay alive?

The longer I spent as a patient the more positive I became that "laying on of the hands" was of paramount importance in the patient-physician relationship. Without a firm, constant, caring physician who will spend the time to look you in the eye, and let you know how much he cares about you and what you are going through, the practice of medicine will be lacking an essential ingredient. The physician must connect with the patient, and to do that he must use all of his senses. He must pick up those vibrations that will allow him to enter into an essential dialogue with the patient. If the patient knows he cares and wants to listen and is not only listening but hearing, then and only then will the patient take a chance and really let the doctor know what he is feeling.

Sometimes, the patient will have reasons for not telling the doctor something and will, if he hears what is being said, tell him so, albeit not directly. I remember when I completed my rotating internship in medicine, which was the year after I graduated medical school, I entered the U.S. Army for a two-year stint. I was commissioned and given the rank of captain. I was sent to Fort Hood, Texas, and became division artillery surgeon in the Second Armored Division. I ran a field dispensary and only served at the Field Hospital as medical officer of the day. My unit was a training unit for new recruits. These recruits came from various parts of the country, often with very little education and often from economically deprived backgrounds. I remember seeing footprints on the toilet seats at times and learned that some of the recruits from backwoods areas had never seen a latrine and were used to going into the woods for a B.M. So they did the same thing by squatting on the toilet seat! This and more faced me and, having just completed my internship, my lack of experience made the task ahead a formidable one.

I remember, one particular Monday morning, one of the recruits came in on sick call complaining of a penile discharge. He particularly emphasized in our discussion that he hadn't been off base and therefore had not had any sexual contact. Remember this was before the time of open admission of homosexuality. But the reason he insisted he hadn't been off base was because he was not allowed off base at that time of his training and if he had told me he was off base he would have had to admit being A.W.O.L. After examining him, I did a gram stain of his urethral discharge and clearly found gram-negative intra-cellular diplococci, confirming my clinical impression of gonorrhea. This posed a real problem. I wanted to treat him appropriately and yet I didn't want to have to make him admit he was off base. By the way, when I told him his diagnosis he stated he must have gotten it from a toilet seat. I then told him I was glad he had told me that because the kind of gonorrhea you got from women was different from the kind you got from toilet seats and now I could give him the right treatment. I then walked out of the room for a few minutes and when I re-entered the room he said, "Doc, maybe you better treat me for the kind you get from women!" The recruit didn't lose face and I didn't try to force him to tell me the truth, and he got the treatment he needed.

June 19 was so much better a day than the day before for me. I knew it during the night because I was much more comfortable. I felt better on mornings like that when I didn't eat, but that wasn't it entirely as I was better when I awakened. I guess that was just one of the vagaries of treatment. Perhaps the sunny day helped also. I had so much more respect for my patients and their symptoms after I had been through this process myself.

Richard Martin, a colleague and legal ethicist/ professor at the Medical College of Georgia, e-mailed me that Brian Carter's dad had died. Brian was a neonatologist in the Children's Medical Center at the Medical College and a bioethicist colleague. I had examined his father the year before at Brian's request when his dad had visited him in Augusta. He had advanced Parkinsonism at that time. I felt badly for Brian as he was in the midst of moving to Nashville to take a position at Vanderbilt and had been trying to close out his position at the Medical College of Georgia, in Augusta, and I believed he had significant unresolved family issues. Like many fathers and sons, too much that needed to be talked about in regard to feelings was never discussed. Brian perhaps had been left with unresolved feelings in regard to his Dad, perhaps some ambivalence that was never dealt with. Now he had had to do it after the fact and that was much more difficult. However, I may have been overstating the case.

As always, I was anxious to finish my Friday treatment and get on the road to Maine. Janet's brother-in-law, Billy, and I were going to try to catch some "stripers"— striped bass, that is. They had made a strong comeback to the tidal waters of Maine and since we were located on one of these tidal waters we would see what we could do. First, we were going to fish for mackerel to be used as bait. I had done this before successfully but never fished for stripers. Billy was a good fisherman and I thought it would be good for him to be thus occupied.

Chapter Seven
GRIEVING FOR MARCIA

Week five of my treatments was beginning and, after returning from Maine that morning, I had my 19th treatment. My trip back that day was marked by considerable urinary urgency. We had to stop twice during the three-hour car ride and I needed to get to my room to void again as soon as I got to Boston. The weekend, as always, was a welcome respite from my treatments and Boston routine. I was glad Billy had been with us. He needed not to be alone on what would have been his and Marcia's 40th wedding anniversary. He was grieving so very much and was in a lot of pain. We looked through his wedding album with him, which was very painful and yet cathartic. He and Janet were able to hold each other and cry and talk about that past life. I did my best to share with them but it was very exhausting for them and for me. I would not have wanted it any other way. I hope Billy will begin to feel less pain and less grief as time goes by. I remember Rabbi Jaffe saying to me, after my 18-year-old daughter, Lori Sue, was killed in an auto accident, that the first year was for grieving but, after that, to continue to grieve was to make a martyr of the loved one who dies and that was not good.

In some ways Billy reminded me of my Uncle Al Berkowitz after my Aunt Ruth died. He was so miserable, couldn't stop crying, was so very lonely and told me he couldn't be alone. He re-married perhaps within a year or so of Aunt Ruth's death, still grieving for her but not able to be alone. I think in his case he needed to do what he did in order to stop grieving. But for Billy, at that time, I think it was just too soon. His grieving and the pain of losing Marcia would have to ease, although I suspect his pain would be with him forever.

I was still having a considerable amount of bowel discomfort and was least uncomfortable when I didn't eat. Saturday I took 5 mg. of prednisone and I think it really helped with the GI distress, although it certainly didn't clear it up. When Jeff called and I told him about taking prednisone, he was upset that I did it on my own without asking my doctor if it was O.K. I suppose he was right, but I had done the same thing with patients enough to know it can help. Having a bowel movement was like defecating through a tight, heavy, narrow tube. Even when finished there was a constant urge to go. Voiding in some ways was similar, but more like passing water through a hot, narrow straw with a heavy surrounding weight around the base of my penis, inside which is particularly heavy at the end of urination.

I was still able to jog and walk for miles and do 50 minutes on my Nordic even though my energy level was a little below my normal. This was a remarkably tiring day and I didn't know why. I did jog in the morning for 40 minutes, had my XRT and then a rather drawn out CT scan of my pelvis at noon primarily for staging purposes prior to the conformal IMRT to start Monday. I had no appetite and ate a soft pretzel at lunch and some egg drop soup and white rice for supper. It sat well, but my degree of fatigue and listlessness was considerable.

The longer I went through this process the more certain I became that one's spirit was of paramount importance in dealing with cancer. You had to never give in to the side effects of the therapy, nor allow yourself the luxury of becoming depressed or feeling sorry for yourself. Your inner strength had to be used. Otherwise the cancer would consume you. I was firmly convinced that this was a spiritual and emotional issue, certainly as much as a physical one. Treatment modalities had improved tremendously and there was certainly more that could be done to prolong life and sustain a better quality of life. But one's state of mind was paramount and I believed much more effort had to be made in dealing with the emotional and spiritual side of cancer treatment.

I awakened the next day feeling much better and was able to jog for 38 minutes before my treatment. My energy level was sub-par but acceptable. Bumped into Philip Reilly, a former acquaintance and sometime business associate, when I was running on the Common and enjoyed seeing him. I hoped we would have lunch or dinner sometime before I leave.

I was having a great deal of difficulty getting to the projects I had planned to do while here. I had planned to begin a monograph on "Medical Ethics for the Patient." I also planned to write and submit an article using the living will of Bill Strong, my close friend, patient and retired pediatric cardiology professor, as the centerpiece. I was also hoping to organize either an Education on Palliative and End-of-Life Care teaching symposium at MCG or arrange to do parts of the EPEC program at various hospitals and/or medical societies in the state. Thus far I had been unable to concentrate sufficiently to do those things. I would have to concentrate on completing my initial plenary session lecture for the beginning of the Phase 1 Ethics program for this year. Being away from home and going through this treatment was incredibly suffocating and oppressive and made working at the same time very difficult. I was keeping up with my e-mail messages. My weekends in Maine were lifesaving, although that previous weekend, grieving with Billy was very fatiguing. Janet continued to be a pillar of strength and love. But, as Lily Tomlin said, "We are all in this together—by ourselves." As each day passed the truth of her statement gained credence.

Janet wrote about this. She said, "Much to my surprise, I feel little need or desire to connect with my family, friends, my usual support system. I feel as though we have left the world that they live in. We no longer have a basis for conversation. I don't know what to talk about. I don't want to talk about anything. I do it only as necessary. In some ways I feel they are all content to have us here in Boston and not be in close touch. Without us in their lives on a daily basis, they can live more normal and less stressful lives. The diagnosis of cancer separates us from all those who have not experienced this. Alan and I seem to exist in some kind of vacuum. We talk to his children and let them tell us how everything is going fine and we agree with whatever they want to hear us say. It is meaningless conversation to us."

"It is hardest for me to talk to Joanie. I can hide nothing from her and my sadness comes bubbling to the surface when I hear her voice. She is always there for me in the most intimate, comfortable way, and all I need is to know that. I don't need much contact. I think I need nothing. I know what I am facing and I just need to get up and see what each day brings and not think about anything beyond that. Whatever I can do to make Alan feel that he is still connected to the world, I want to do. I think perhaps he might feel as disconnected as I and I don't want him feeling disconnected from me, too."

Joanie, our good friend, had sent me five stones, each with a particular quality that was supposedly beneficial in cases of illness. One of the stones was a small, irregular piece of light brown zircite that was supposed to help heal the prostate. It is amazing to me how we grasp for anything that might help. Such feelings undoubtedly go back to the days of witchcraft and icons and folklore. I think we are willing to accept all the help we can get no matter how illogical or whimsical it is. I believe this is one of the reasons alternative medicine has become so popular.

June 17, 1999, was a day that was entirely energyless for me. I did jog in the morning but, after that, walking to our post office and being on my feet was a great effort. I took a long nap in the afternoon, but never regained my energy and felt tired and listless all day. I finally went to sleep and really didn't awaken except to go to the bathroom two or three times until 8:20 the next morning, which was a good 10 or 11 hours of sleep. For me that was incredible. I awakened, felt somewhat rested, still without appetite but thirsty, drank some apple and cranberry juice, took my 23rd treatment and headed out to the airport to pick up Jeff and Ally.

I completed treatment #25 the following day, which ended the conventional external beam radiation treatment. The day after would begin the conformal intensity modulated radiotherapy (IMRT). This required a trans-abdominal ultrasound before each treatment to identify the exact location of the prostate. A computerized construct of my prostate would allow for maximum radiation to be delivered primarily to the prostate itself. I would also receive another anti-androgen injection, which meant another three months of being a eunuch. There were no really good five- or ten-year cancer-free survival statistics yet for this combined therapy, so only time would tell. Whatever I believed, not being able to make love to my wife was a high price to pay

I hated being impotent probably more than anything else involved in this ordeal but I did want to live as long as I could, as long as my quality of life was good. What a conflict within myself. I wanted to make love to my wife desperately and as soon as possible, and yet I wanted to stay with her as long as possible. It was strange how one learned to settle in this situation. What you thought you couldn't tolerate became tolerable when you knew it might be life-prolonging.

Chapter Eight

JEFF, ALLY AND MAINE

My son, Jeff and 15-month-old granddaughter, Ally, were with us for the last weekend of June, spending the first night at the Neely House. There, Ally played with a two-year-old blind child from the Philippines, here for treatment of a malignant tumor. The treatment that is keeping her alive has cost her her eyesight. What a contrast, the healthy and just-beginning life, and the just-beginning but dying life.

Jeff and I cut wood for the woodstove and dug clams and jogged the hills for 53 minutes. When we returned home and I saw Janet I could only hold her and cry tears of joy mixed with sadness. I cannot stress enough how important it is to keep your spirits high when you have a life-threatening illness or are receiving stressful treatment. Do not, under any circumstance give up or think every symptom or side effect is the end.

July 1's treatment left me with six more to go. After the following day's treatment I was to leave for Maine for the long July 4 weekend. I couldn't wait. Dan Rahn and family, plus one child-friend of their children, would be in Friendship at a B&B for the last two days of their vacation, Sunday and Monday. We didn't have room for them in our small house but I was looking forward to spending time with them and showing them a bit of our Maine environs.

I seemed to be having more urinary symptoms with the conformal IMRT and was waiting for the GI symptoms to subside, which hadn't happened yet. It was sort of like being nauseated and hungry at the same time. Also, I didn't have too much energy that day. It did seem like my symptoms were worse toward the middle of the week. There probably was a psychological component, but also perhaps the effects built up as the week progressed, after not having treatments on the weekend. The main thing was to keep going and not let my spirits deteriorate.

Our friend, Andy H. was having a helluva time in Atlanta, and we had been peripherally involved as Karen (Janet's older sister, living in Atlanta) was so close to them, and kept calling to get my input and keep us abreast of what was going on. To summarize, Andy was 60 years old and had obstructive jaundice, probably due to an ampullary carcinoma. Unfortunately they could not do ERCP because of a large paraesophageal hernia, so a transhepatic cholangiogram was done which revealed a mass near the head of the pancreas. A stent was placed and removed today, followed by a spiking fever suggesting ascending cholangitis. (All of this was secondhand via Karen). In any case, I discussed the situation with my friends, Joe Griffin at MCG and Nordy Greenberger at the University of Kansas, (both excellent gastroenterologists with much experience). They mentioned two doctors, one at Hopkins, one at Mass General, both excellent physicians with much experience with pancreatic and ampullary cancers. However, I thought Andy was too sick to move, wanted to stay in Atlanta and would probably have surgery there. In any case this was a real bummer. It didn't seem as if anyone was free of their own grief, but as difficult as it was, I would not want to have been deprived of contributing my input, for whatever it was worth.

While I was writing this, I could hear Janet's side of a phone call with her Mom. She was telling her that my treatments were almost completed, and then responded to something her Mom said by saying, "Oh no, we won't know for a long time what the results will be." And so it went. There was no crystal ball. This wasn't like a sonogram in pregnancy to definitely tell the mother the sex of the child. I could only hope and pray for a long remission

Chapter Nine
THE PATIENT-PHYSICIAN RELATIONSHIP

My treatments were winding down. This cancer thing was all-pervasive and the treatment sucked me into a very uncomfortable frame of mind. For others undergoing similar experiences, I must warn you not to give in to it. There will be side effects, loss of energy, increased fatigue. You must resist giving in. I would advise having the treatments where you live, if possible. I want to say once again how important it is for patients to have the compassion and empathy of their physicians; their own personal internist or family practitioner, as well as the specialists and sub-specialists involved in their treatment and care.

I cannot help but mention my philosophy of how medicine and our culture has changed over the last few decades. We have become a nation of catchphrases and keywords. Our vocabulary is increasingly full of jargon. Now we have "user-friendly" and "pre-owned cars" and patients as "clients," to mention a few. But what is fundamentally flawed is the designation "primary care physician." Captured in this phrase is a philosophy that embodies a fatal flaw in the perception of what a physician is. Because of this designation all internists without a sub-specialty are now primary care physicians. They are lumped with family medicine docs and pediatricians. That means that someone like me, with 35 years of practice experience, who grew up when we didn't have intensivists, and who was the intensivist, for all practical purposes, but who also had a private practice in internal medicine, is now a primary care physician. It doesn't matter that I am now, and have been for the last 17 years, an associate professor of medicine at a medical school, teaching medical students and residents how to practice medicine by caring for patients in the inpatient as well as ambulatory arena. It doesn't matter that I am certified by the American Board of Internal Medicine and re-certified by that same board, and elected a Fellow in the American College of Physicians and given Added Qualifications in Geriatric Medicine by the American Board of Internal Medicine (although I choose not to exclusively practice geriatric medicine). Nevertheless, because of our "catchphrase" mentality and our managed care vocabulary I am a primary care physician.

Why does this designation so incense me? It does so because it changes the expectations of the patients and those residents in internal medicine who will complete their training in general internal medicine and will go out into private practice as primary care physicians. They will have been taught the essentials of general internal medicine but will also have been taught that if they face a medical problem they can always call the sub-specialist for help. This will inherently lead to these physicians feeling secure in not knowing many things they should know because the specialist will know. They will be viewed by their patients in that light as well, and be seen more as a way station, as a triage physician, someone capable of taking care of non-life threatening illness such as respiratory infections or urinary tract infections and such, and someone who will refer serious problems to a specialist. The other side of the coin is just as deadly, in that the internist will view himself as a primary caregiver and will not maintain what skills he has been taught in his training program, since he will not be viewed by his patients or the insurance community or medical community, for that matter, as having those skills.

What are some of the serious consequences of this development? I will give you examples of two:

Our emergency rooms are over-used and over-worked. To put this into perspective, in 2005, there were 110 million emergency room visits in the United States. One of the reasons is the primary care physician mentality, although there are other factors: the number of uninsured and the EMTALA Act, which does not allow patients to be turned away from the emergency departments, as well as the unavailability of enough general internists. No longer does the physician have to go to the emergency room to meet and assess his patient. No, the E.R. doc can evaluate and begin treatment and admit, or treat and discharge. The internist can effectively become the triage physician, or "way station" if you will.

In fact, more often than not the personal physician is not involved. As an example, my wife's 85-year old step-dad developed a severe respiratory infection. He is a diabetic and rapidly became dehydrated with poor fluid intake, a fever, and underlying marginal fluid balance. He became so weak that he could not stand without someone holding him. When his primary care physician was called, a nurse answered the call. The nurse, covering for several doctors, stated since he wasn't one of her patients she could only tell him to take Robitussin or go to the emergency room. His physician, therefore, was already out of the loop.

After eight hours in the emergency room he was admitted for further care. Eight hours when his physician could have perhaps assessed the situation over the phone and decided what his patient needed. If he decided the patient needed to be seen he could have met him in the emergency room, notified the E.R. he was on the way, evaluated the patient within the hour, saved an eight-hour wait and the expense of emergency room care. Moreover, the patient and family would have had a chance to find out what their physician thought was wrong and what he intended to do. In other words the patient-physician relationship would have been activated and the family given the reassurance they needed.

Instead the family left the hospital at midnight, after eight hours still not knowing what was wrong with their family member and obligated to wait until the following morning for a report. Let me assure you that this occurred in a large metropolitan hospital in Atlanta, Georgia, and I would guess that this same scenario is being re-enacted in many hospitals throughout the land. I believe part of the responsibility for this abrogation of physician responsibility rests with the transition from a fee-for-service system to what is now a mixed bag, and where the primary care physician designation becomes the modus operandi. We now have primary care physicians, specialists, intensivists, and now hospitalists! That essential patient-physician bond is being eroded by a mindset, by a way of practicing medicine, by insurance-run health care, and by a philosophy of health care delivery that is inherently wrong.

Let me give you a second example of the fallacy of our developing health care system. One week before my wife's step-dad became ill, his primary care provider, as he is also called, ran a battery of blood tests. One of the tests showed an elevated alkaline phosphatase. The next we heard, he had a hepatitis profile and was told he might have hepatitis A and/or B. He was then scheduled for a CT scan of his abdomen and an appointment made with a gastroenterologist. Reviewing this sequence of events, I can only assume his doctor is ordering tests and doesn't know what to do with abnormal test results. Furthermore, I believe he has been taught that a specialist can figure out what is wrong. He doesn't need to know that ordering a gamma GT blood test may help differentiate liver alkaline phosphatase from bone alkaline phosphatase. He doesn't need to know that a hepatitis A antibody may only mean past illness and that many of us carry this antibody. He doesn't need to know the difference between an IgG and IgM antibody. And so on. Of course, the mind-set is that the specialist can piece it all together.

What can we do to alter this pathway down which we are being propelled? First, I believe we must change our mind-set and stop thinking of general internists as gatekeepers and way stations and primary care physicians. We must train our Internal medicine residents to be specialists in general internal medicine, not only in practice but in spirit as well. We must instill in them the absolute knowledge that they are responsible for their patients whether they are in the Emergency Room or at home or in the hospital.

Second, the public must be educated that their general internist is a specialist who can take care of the vast majority of medical problems that arise. Third, it is essential that physicians take back much of the responsibility of patient communication from the office staff, nurse practitioner or answering service. The patient must have access to his physician. At this point in time, it is as if the physician's office staff is running interference for him. This won't change unless physicians are willing to make it change and unless patients refuse to accept this state of health care delivery. My worry is that the more patients and physicians are raised in this milieu, the fewer will be the number of physicians and patients who know how it used to be. Eventually, those who did will have forgotten or be gone, and what we now see will be taken for granted.

Chapter Ten

MY JANET

July 8 saw one more treatment to go, yahoo, one more treatment to go. As hard as the beginning of all this was, the end was equally difficult. The last week seemed to be an interminable one but the next day would be the last of this phase. Sitting in the radiation oncology waiting room that morning with the other patients was a most poignant experience. The conversation at first had to do with the remarkable qualities of Abby, the two-year-old with retinoblastoma, undergoing radiation after the surgical removal of both eyes. Abby was put to sleep before each treatment so all in the waiting room saw her coming in awake and going out asleep. And Abby had the blessing of childhood resilience and curiosity and forbearance.

Abby would come up to you and feel your arm or your leg and then ask, "What's your name?" Although Filipino, she was very much bilingual. She went up to one of the women patients that morning and felt her purse and asked, "What is that"? When told by the woman it was her purse Abby commented, because of its size, "Big money!" Her courage and spirit were remarkable and, mixed with sadness, were a boost to everyone's morale. That morning, one of the women patients with head and neck cancer had been talking about the camaraderie of the patients and their families and the lack of any hostility. We all felt that, I think. And everyone knew what everyone had and shared the good and bad. They were truly pleased when someone was finishing their treatment or had a good report. One of the women was receiving chemotherapy for what sounded like small cell cancer of the lung. She was getting cisplatin and taxol and announced to the group of waiting patients that she was told the tumor had completely disappeared. Everyone expressed their good wishes and joked a bit about her baldness. All in all, I believed these patients were doing their own group therapy. Perhaps such sessions should be part of the treatment for all cancer patients. I would even suggest having a cancer patient be the facilitator.

I was very irritable and sad that entire week. It was an effort to go back for treatment after the long weekend in Maine. I had not been able to accomplish very much, work-wise, during my treatment. I suspected the effort to concentrate was too much for me. Hopefully that would change once I left there.

I want to say once again how important it is for patients to have the compassion and empathy of their physicians. Too many of us physicians are not caring, feeling, sensitive human beings. I know now, if I never knew before, why I insisted on maintaining control of my patients. They never had to forego the tender, loving care they needed. The surgeon could do his thing and I was always there, pre- and post-operatively, to minister to, lay on the hands, to explain what was going on, interpret for the patient; always willing and needing to be demanding of the specialists, and holding them accountable. They didn't have carte blanche with my patients.

I remember one surgeon who was doing a cholecystectomy on one of my patients and after the surgery called me to tell me that he had decided to repair a hiatal hernia while in there. This was without the patient's consent or mine for that matter. This was, I thought, inappropriate, told him so and never used him again. The physicians who worked with me understood what I demanded of them, respected me for caring and for demanding the best even if they would have preferred for me to just agree with whatever they were doing. I have even gone into the operating room and watched over the surgeon's shoulder at times. This is a wonderful way to see how a surgeon handles himself under stress, his judgment, how he deals with the operating room personnel, and so on. This is a very good way to see how the surgeon handles "tissue." A gentle surgeon is a good surgeon. I am very sad to see health care delivery systems that don't allow for this essential of the patient-physician relationship. I will continue in my training of students and house staff to emphasize the importance of humanism in the practice of medicine. Bernard Lown has made a similar point quite eloquently in his book "The Lost Art of Healing." I fear he is, unfortunately, too right.

Chapter Eleven
FAREWELL TO THE NEELY HOUSE

My last and final radiation treatment was on July 9. When I was taking my last walk down the hallway in the Neely House, leaving my residence quarters for the last time and heading down for my last radiation oncology appointment, I burst into tears. The sheer completion of this time at the New England Medical Center suddenly left me feeling overwhelmed: a sense of, what do I do now? I cannot describe the stresses involved in going through these treatments away from home and with this life-threatening illness.

We left for Maine right after my last radiation treatment. I had been having trouble with my right eye misting over in a small quadrant of my visual field. This had occurred sporadically for several months and I finally saw the ophthalmologist at NEMC. He found nothing wrong with my vision and no cataracts or retinal problem or abnormal pressure. He thought it could have been an ophthalmic migraine equivalent! Well, whatever it was, it didn't occur once during the week after I left Boston. Perhaps it was stress-induced vascular migraine effects. Could I have been under such stress without knowing it? Of course I could have, and was, and did know it. I still felt stressed and uncertain of the future, but at least the ordeal of my stay at NEMC and conformal IMRT was over and I was in Maine where I felt so blessed to have been given that safe haven to recuperate in.

Going through cancer treatment can become your life. That is, you can allow the illness itself to become your life. You must guard against this if at all possible. The week after leaving Boston was a true Godsend, but not without a continuing emotional rollercoaster ride. My physical complaints following radiation had not subsided as yet, both urinary and GI, and my hot flashes persisted as well. Needless to say my impotence continued.

For those of you who have to go through this kind of business, you need to do it with my Janet, or rather your Janet. Our relationship continued and continues, to amaze me. At the expense of sounding trite and corny, Janet, is, in every way, my love, my friend, my counselor. I cannot describe the wonder and depth of what we have together.

One morning in Maine, Janet and I were talking about my anger with the computer's functionality, and my having to depend upon her to help me. It was hard for me to accept the fact that I was computer-ignorant, but I knew it to be so. This opened up an overwhelming sadness for me and I realized how inadequate I was feeling and how having to depend upon her so much was so degrading to me. And, of course my inability to have a continuing sexual relationship with Janet was most humiliating and demoralizing. The radiation and anti-androgen treatment had other less occult effects as well. For instance, my pubic hair had become quite sparse and the underarm hair seemed sparse and not growing normally, as well. I believed my skin texture and body odor were different. I was uncertain my body contours were different but I imagined that I was rounder and softer. This may have been my imagination. I certainly had not had any obvious breast development, although I kept looking for it.

I did believe my strength was to some degree less, as was my energy, but I could still do a good deal. I noticed the difference in strength playing tennis, where my serve and other strokes had less pace and my endurance or stamina was off a bit. I think being physically fit has been a life's work for me. I have compulsively attempted to maintain my physical well-being. I am certain getting old is more difficult for some than others. For me the fact that Janet is 16 years younger than I am was a major stimulus to keep me functioning at a high level. I perhaps should have been 10 years younger, and the disparity in our ages less significant. But this was one of the reasons I continued with my exercise program faithfully. I still ran or did my Nordic every day, and for 50 minutes more or less covering three to five miles. Then a full day's work, followed by a tennis match three times a week.

I often then cooked dinner, did some reading and, under ordinary circumstances, had enough left to make love to my wife several times a week or more. The funny thing was that now, although very rare with my anti-androgen treatment, I was still able to have an erection. One night when I was so sad, Janet and I discussed some of my fears. I let her know how inadequate I felt in so many ways, with my dependency upon her carrying over into making decisions, feeling in some ways child-like in my dependency needs. Well, after all that crying and talk, we were hugging and suddenly I was aware of an erection that was sufficient to have intercourse! What a wonderful surprise. To feel Janet again that way was absolutely fulfilling, even without the ability to have an orgasm. I could only look heavenward and say, "Thank you,God." I felt it was a clear message from God and one I need to remember and be thankful for. There is a God and he was watching over me and letting me know this.

Chapter Twelve
MOOD SWINGS

Why did my mood fluctuate so? I was becoming irritable, nervous, tough to live with. I had lost my self-esteem, had become too dependent on Janet and felt resentful about it. I seemed to have put Janet in a no-win situation. I asked her to be responsible for things and then resented her for doing so. We were so close, perhaps too close, and everything hurt. We were so close and yet, in some ways, not close enough. Without question, my eunuch state had a great deal to do with my mood.

We had gone through so much and yet I didn't know if my treatments had been successful. What would happen when I stopped the anti-androgens? Would I regain my sexual potency, would the cancer recur, and would I have to go back on the chemical castration? Would that keep the cancer in check? These were questions without answers. In the meantime, we had to get back to our normal existence, back to work. The physical side effects of the radiation were of little matter to me, except for the impotence. I did resent having to be impotent to perhaps stay alive. Janet and I would do better at home, as good as this time in Maine had been. I thanked God for Janet and our love.

We were beginning to close up the house in preparation for our return to Augusta. I would miss my Maine retreat. As much as I wanted to get back to work, I had mixed feelings about leaving this "safe haven." I had lost a great deal of my self-confidence and self-esteem. Whether my being impotent should have been so significant to me or not, it just was, and all stemmed from that, as well as from having cancer. I cannot explain how these two issues were so devastating to my sense of wellbeing and self-assuredness. I was hoping that, when I got over the side effects of my treatment and got back to productive work, my outlook would change. I can only urge all those patients with cancer and secondary side effects of therapy never to give up what they have been doing in terms of their routines and, particularly, not to stop working. I hope their work is as satisfying to them as mine is to me. I believe it to be a major part of my ego strength and can only assume others are in a similar position. If I had to say what I think are the most important ingredients in surviving cancer and its treatment, it would be the following:

- Keep working if at all possible.
- Work at your love relationship and don't distance yourself from your spouse. Love is essential to the healing process.

- Have faith in God, or whatever you accept as the controlling force in your existence. Never lose that faith and acceptance of your ultimate destiny.
- Maintain a sense of humor. There is humor in even the most devastating events of life.
- Life is a circle with a beginning and an end. Believe and know "what goes around comes around."
- And, remember Lily Tomlin's words: "We are all in this together—by ourselves."

My woodpile in the basement was now replenished, all wood having been cut and split and stored indoors. A lot of work, but also a lot of fun and a real sense of accomplishment, knowing that I would have adequate wood for the wood stove through the rest of that year for our infrequent visits. Naturally, there was often a price to pay for all this labor, namely my arms were constantly scraped and black-and-blue from the bruises I incurred, and particularly from carrying the wood into the basement. On top of that I had dropped a log on my little toe four days before and this was the first day I had been able to wear a shoe. The toe doubled in size, became totally black-and-blue, and made me think I had probably chipped a bone. I neglected to put ice on it when it happened and my taking aspirin made everything get more bloody-looking. This had really interfered with my exercise, as I was unable to jog or go for walks.

Fortunately I had my Nordic and had continued doing 50 minutes every day, as well as my wood- cutting and multiple other chores, including clamming. Clamming is a very interesting, intriguing, and satisfying endeavor. At low tide, since we were on tidal water, I could walk out to the shoals and harvest mussels without any effort, as they were on the surface. The clams had to be dug with a clamming rake or fork, which is a six-pronged pitchfork bent at more than a 90 degree angle, with the wooden handle cut to about 18 to 24 inches. You had to get deep enough to get the clams and look for holes in the muck indicating a clam beneath the surface. It was hard work, but what a pleasure to sit down to a bucket of fresh steamers that you had harvested yourself hours before steaming. These were soft-shell clams and were good primarily for steaming or using in chowder. So I had kept very busy. We had had to haul our boat, moored in deep water in back of our house, onto its trailer and into Rockland Marine to have it pressure-washed and engine-serviced. We would pick it up that day and trailer it back to Augusta tomorrow. The canoe and dinghy had to be stored in our basement after being cleaned by me, and the 2 H.P. Johnson winterized, flushed out, etc. for winter storage. Closing up our house was labor-intensive. Thank God we had the strength and wherewithal to do it.

I would miss this Maine retreat but I had needed this respite and felt almost ready to resume normal life and work. I say almost because I am not a very optimistic person and have misgivings and hesitancy about any change, and we certainly had had change those last few months.

Chapter Thirteen
CHEMICAL CASTRATION

Our friends Alan and Donna Podis left July 31 after a three-day visit. I had great respect for Alan's knowledge of urology and would forever be grateful to him for leading me through the maze of medical decision-making related to having prostate cancer. However I was glad they were gone and Janet and I had our small home in the woods to ourselves. I am not very gregarious and I value my privacy. In some ways I have always considered myself a misanthrope. I am just more comfortable alone and with Janet. We just seem to fit into each other, like one of those interlocking puzzles. I don't seem to need anything or anyone else.

I am very routinized and used to doing things my way. I like having my routines and, as I grew older, I think I was becoming less interested in changes. Besides that, I was so much more aware of my finiteness, my mortality, since knowing and being treated for cancer.

I wanted every moment to be the way I wanted it to be. There was so much more I wanted to do and I doubted there would be enough time. I wanted more of Janet, too. I never had enough of her. It wasn't that way without testosterone. My head said it wasn't any different but my entire being didn't feel it the same way at all. Not ever feeling horny was a terrible way to live. The inability to physically perform was the smaller part of the loss. Not wanting Janet sexually—not wanting to smell her hair, to kiss her mouth, to want to feel her close to me, to feel that stirring inside—that was the greater loss by far, and one I never appreciated as a physician, nor, for that matter as a person. That was a loss that Viagra can never replace. A man needs his testosterone.

It had been 10 months since my prostate cancer was diagnosed. It had also been 10 months since my chemical castration. I don't think any physician, and I include myself in the years before I had cancer, has the foggiest notion of what chemical castration does to a man. More than that, I don't think most doctors really want to know. Before my testosterone was taken away my life revolved around three essential elements. Number one was my passion and love for my wife. Number two was my tennis and my jogging. Number three was my work. After losing testosterone everything changes.

The night our friends left we made love, Janet and I. Our lovemaking was different now, partly because of physical limitations imposed by the year with complete androgen blockade, partly by the side effects of the radiation treatments, which included no ejaculate with orgasm, and an inability to achieve a full erection, and partly because of both Janet's and my own emotional response to my cancer and to the effects of the treatment. You see, we both approached the physical changes differently. Janet and I talked about this recently as we drove to Boothbay Harbor to pick up some needlepoint thread Janet needed. I have to tell you that having gone through my cancer treatment had made my physical capabilities, sexually, much more uncertain. I didn't know at all times how and whether my body parts would function. This made me much more tentative, and, as Janet told me, made her much more tentative also. It was sometimes like we were tap-dancing around each other, both wanting the same thing but not wanting to hurt each other's feelings, and, for me, wanting to avoid that feeling of humiliation that came with inability to perform.

But it was so much more than that. I need to tell you of the physical limitations but most of all I have to tell you how absolutely wonderful and exciting it is to want Janet the way I do now, the way I couldn't without my testosterone. That feeling, that desire, that horniness, that heightened inner excitement of wanting my wife, my lover, so far transcends the physical deficiencies that there is no comparison. Thank God, I feel Janet again; no, my erection isn't as hard as it used to be; no, I can't always maintain an erection; no, my certainty that I won't suddenly lose the erection no longer exists; no, that sudden surge of blood flow into my penis when I am inside my wife with the rush of intensified feeling, of being able to feel her so much more fully, is no longer possible; and now, the orgasm that seems much more quixotic and less under my control, but yet still so wonderful; yet, now without ejaculation which the radiation treatments have deprived me of; yes, these changes have occurred but lovemaking with my love, my Janet is and will always be, wonderful, exhilarating.

Having said all that, we had both become so tentative, not knowing, for Janet, what I wanted and what I was capable of at any given moment, and me not knowing really what she was feeling and wanting, afraid, almost, both of us, to commit to our lovemaking. So our foreplay was so much less, so much less exciting. It was as if we are both saying, let's get this lovemaking over with while maybe we can. Do it, but, well, don't get too worked up just in case. At least I think that was what we are thinking. One of the complexities of this entire issue was how little we knew of what the other was feeling. Janet and I were blessed with a love and a comfort level that allowed us to explore our feelings together, in words. Even then, how much of each other's feelings did we comprehend? And how did this equate with other couples going through a similar catastrophic life event? All I can say is, keep talking, keep communicating, don't ever cut yourself off from your love, don't distance yourself from your mate, don't stop sharing anything, and don't ever presume to know what the other is feeling. You have to ask and maybe you will know some of what the other is going through.

August second, I wrote in my journal "EXTRA! EXTRA! EXTRA! Orgasm without Ejaculation Comes to Friendship, Maine!" Why should I think that warrants front-page news? Only because it is probably happening in thousands of homes throughout the world, where there are men who have been treated with radiotherapy for prostate cancer and who have not been told of this consequence of the treatment. Absence of ejaculate, which means absence of semen with orgasm, also occurs after a TURP, or transurethral resection of the prostate for benign enlargement of the prostate that may be causing obstruction to the flow of urine. In this latter case, there is retrograde ejaculation, which means the ejaculate goes backward rather than forward, and, therefore, doesn't come out. As Jimmy Durante might have said, 'What a revoltin' development!' "

The question is, isn't this something physicians should routinely discuss with their patients? From this patient's viewpoint (mine, that is), it certainly should be. In contrast to transurethral resection of the prostate for benign enlargement, absence of semen at orgasm in prostate cancer is a consequence of radiation therapy, and, yet, if not for my urologist friend who had his prostate cancer radiotherapy a few months before mine and who mentioned this in passing, I would not have been aware of this eventuality. True, this is a small matter in the overall scheme of things, but still something that helps if you know of it and can incorporate it into your thinking. What is that expression, "Forewarned is forearmed"? A small thing, yes, but yet another small insult to add to the myriad of other small insults; and just as troublesome to physicians who are patients as to those with no medical knowledge. All those small insults do add up.

But, I thanked God for the ability to have an orgasm with my wife, with or without ejaculation. No, more than that, I thanked God for giving me the desire to have an orgasm with my wife. I thanked God for giving me back my testosterone for however long. The wanting was so much more important than the doing, at least to me. Yet, darn it, it was important to me. Don't ask me why. Was it ego? Was it a macho thing? Was it just the testosterone talking? Well, I guess a little of each, but the bottom line was: it made me feel like a man.

We were packing and would leave for Augusta and home in the morning. Our stay this time had been wonderful. I had been able to happily perform what I called my four essential activities: jogging; playing tennis (and winning); making love to my wife; using my brain—and not necessarily in that order. But, of utmost importance, was the closeness I continued to feel for Janet. She has truly been my salvation, my strength, my love, my passion, my friend and, in many ways, my super-ego. I counted my blessings. I considered myself rich, indeed, loving Janet and having her love in return. In the Talmud, it is asked, "Who is rich?" It answers, "He who rejoices in what he has." (The Talmud Midrash Avot 4:1.) Amen to that.

Chapter Fourteen

BREAST SORENESS, HOT FLASHES, FORMER PATIENTS

The day came when I slept through the night and, when I awakened, I realized that I had no breast or nipple soreness for the first time since my treatments. I was able to turn over, sleep on my front without feeling any discomfort. Janet, I remembered, at times had breast tenderness, usually at certain times during her menstrual cycle. Until I had the same thing I never really appreciated what it was like. Just like the hot flashes. I had no idea what that was like until I started having them. Those weren't things you learned in medical school, or even practicing medicine for that matter. I guess it takes one to know one! What a pleasure to turn over in bed and not feel breast soreness. My breasts were bigger since my chemical castration and had not felt "normal" until this week. I knew they would never fully regain their previous size and shape, but that I could put up with. What with my exercise and my lifting weights, my body habitus wasn't too far from what it was before anti-androgens. The 20 pounds I had gained when taking anti-androgens had pretty much been lost.

We were back in Maine for a few weeks. I had many thoughts about cancer and how to approach living with cancer. I have to tell you about my former patients, the Millers, and how Jerry's stroke told me something about what I might be willing to endure when my cancer recurs. I will also tell you about androgen blockade, taking care of other physicians, living with the uncertainty of my PSA level and not letting this uncertainty run my life, and about several patients I now take care of and what they have taught me.

It was now 13 months since my last anti-androgen treatment and that injection was a three-month depot shot so I had been off anti-androgens for about nine months, although there may have been a gradually reducing and lingering effect. I was not totally back to my previous level. My self-confidence, my libido, my feeling of manliness, my aggressiveness was still off the mark and probably always would be. I didn't know whether I would need anti-androgens again, but dreaded the thought. I was not the same person without my testosterone. There was fat in places fat never was before. My muscles weren't as taut. My sexual desire was blunted. When I was playing competitive tennis and the score was tied, invariably I lost because I was not able to raise my level of play a notch as I could have before. When I looked at Janet the juices flowed, but not as fully as before. That initial anticipatory excitement was not as acute. Amazing how important testosterone was.

It had been not quite a year since my last radiotherapy treatment and I was to have another PSA at one year to assess, if possible, whether my cancer seemed to be controlled. I was afraid to get the test. I almost didn't want to know. Would it be very low, let's say 0.2 or less? Or would it be 0.3 as it was three months ago? Or would it be higher, suggesting recurrence or activity of the cancer? I would get the PSA done, perhaps next week.

As I looked out on the tide coming in and felt the rain fast approaching I could not help but think back to a little over one year before, when I had sat in the same place looking out on Meduncook River inlet on which my house was located. We were packing up then and heading back to Augusta and home after completing the radiation treatments. We were no more certain of our future then than we were now. That is one thing about having cancer. You just never know what lies ahead except the certainty that sometime, in some way, the cancer will be back. Whether you have symptoms right now or not, cancer rarely lets go. That certainty is with you every moment of every day and probably when you are sleeping as well, rolling around in your subconscious somewhere. It is truly all-pervasive. But go on you must, and should. You still must take every day as a new day, for it is all any of us have, with or without cancer. Nobody said life was easy. I have often told my older patients, faced with one infirmity or another and not happy about it, that getting old is not for sissies.

We don't get to choose what God gives us but we do get to decide how we come to terms with it. I have to tell you about my daughter, Lori, and after I do you will know why I do so at this point, in talking about cancer always being with me.

Lori was my youngest child and my only daughter . . .

I have to tell you that several hours have gone by since I started to tell you about Lori. That is because I started to sob uncontrollably and couldn't go on. It has been that way ever since Lori died. Certain painful events in one's life never go away.

Lori was 18 years old in 1981 when she was killed in a head-on collision while sitting in the front passenger seat of a Volkswagen Sirocco, coming back on Alligator Alley from Sanibel Island in South Florida with another couple and a boyfriend. The two boys survived and the two girls were killed instantly. I don't remember the mile-marker. Perhaps I don't want to remember, but I did, years after her death, go to that mile-marker with Janet, hoping to find some kind of something. What is it called nowadays? Closure? You see, we have words for everything but nothing describes the feelings; not in my book, anyway.

It took me years before I could even attempt to go to that mile-marker. I had not been on Alligator Alley from the time Lori died to that day. I have not been there since, nor will I ever go there again. Just thinking of Alligator Alley, I break out in a cold sweat. When Lori died, I was living alone in an apartment on Sheridan Street in Hollywood, Florida. Sue, my first wife, and I, were separated and in the process of getting a divorce. Lori, confused, mixed-up kid that she was, at age 18, living at home with Sue, was the love of my life. It wasn't just the divorce that caused her to be mixed-up and confused. It really followed a very turbulent adolescence from which I doubt she ever fully recovered.

Losing her was, without question, the most painful event ever, for me; and yes, there was guilt and hurt and so much else besides my love for her. The pain of loss seemed unbearable and I questioned how I could go on. In my grief I even debated going back to Lori's mother. It was as if losing a child and losing a wife at the same time was too much to bear. But what I wanted to say was that the pain of losing her, of losing a child, never goes away. Yes, it became less oppressive but never, ever left. Not a day has gone by since her death that I haven't thought of her. The years multiply but the pain of losing her is always there. If I meet someone named Lori, I cannot say her name. And so it is with having cancer. It never leaves you. I hear people who have cancer talking about being survivors. I don't see that. What have they survived? The initial treatment, a remission perhaps? But they still have cancer, as do I. The cancer is still in you, albeit under some kind of control. Every day you wonder when it will manifest itself again, knowing that it will, in time. You have survived for now. If you are an optimist you are a survivor, and if a pessimist (or a realist?) you are a victim. I am a pessimist.

When Janet and I were out walking we passed an old farmhouse with the name of Miller out front. That reminded me of a former patient named J. Miller. He and his wife, Hannah, retired to Florida from New York City. They were two delightful people, in their mid-sixties, very much in love and kind to one other. It was a pleasure taking care of them medically. Until J. had a big stroke

leaving him paralyzed on one side—hemiplegic—and
with an expressive aphasia. He knew what he wanted to
say but couldn't get it to come out right. And every time
he came to my office and I looked him in the eye and
we started to talk about how he was feeling, he started
to cry. Some of his crying may have been involuntary
and secondary to post-stroke emotional lability, but
most was a realistic sadness and frustration and anger
because of his limitations. Yes, he was depressed and
why shouldn't he be, with such a sudden, devastating
and debilitating traumatic illness? He knew he would
never again be the way he had been before the stroke,
that is, a vibrant, healthy man. Nothing we talked about,
no encouragement on my part, no amount of physical
therapy and rehabilitation—including a time in the
Rusk Institute in New York—changed his physical and
speech limitations, nor his outlook.

I could do so little for him, or for his wife, except to be
there for them, to sit and listen, to care about them and
share in a small way what they were both going through.
He was so miserable and Hannah tried to stay as upbeat
as possible. Not a whole lot different from what Janet
and I were going through, at least emotionally. What I
could give him was so inadequate because what he had
to come to terms with was, to him, an insurmountable
obstacle. It was, in fact, that devastating. Thankfully he
died of another stroke two years later without additional
suffering.

I guess I felt that, if my cancer became as limiting
as J's stroke, I would think about using that syringe
full of morphine. Janet had made me promise not to
do anything without her knowing. That made it very

difficult. But I would not be Morrie, of "Tuesdays with Morrie," with amyotrophic lateral sclerosis—Lou Gehrig's Disease—who feared only the indignity of not being able to wipe himself after a bowel movement.

My urologist friend was visiting for the weekend and it occurred to me, after I saw him, that I had not written to him with the results of my last PSA, which had been done the week before I left for Maine. It took me several weeks to get up enough courage to get the PSA. This was three months after my last one, which was 0.3 and which was obtained when I had been off anti-androgen treatment for six months. The 0.3 was good, I thought.

Finally, on July 10, 2000, I had a repeat PSA done. You see, that is one of the problems of being a physician. No one tells me what to do. I get a PSA when I want to. Oh, sure, my friend Alan Podis told me to get one around then but, no visit to the doctor, no reminder from the doctor's office—just me deciding to do it! Physicians, even your own physician, leave their physician patients alone. Why is that? Do we think physicians can make their own decisions about their illness? Do we, as physicians, feel intimidated by other physicians? I care for many physicians in my practice and over the years, have realized that taking care of other physicians should be a specialty in its own right. We could call it "physician colleague medicine." I do believe it requires much that is different from caring for non-physician patients. Of paramount importance in being a physician's physician is having complete confidence in your ability to fill that role. Well, maybe more about this later.

Getting back to my PSA, it was 0.3. That meant there was no indication that the cancer was becoming active again. So that was good, and what a relief. I did not expect it to be lower, but what if it was higher? What if the results suggested I needed anti-androgen treatment again to try to control the cancer that was roaring back? Would I have been willing to undergo it? I don't know. But what a way to live, waiting for the next PSA! I was a prisoner of a blood test! Is that how I would live out the rest of my days, waiting for the next PSA? I guess that is a choice I could make. I could decide if I wanted to live that way or not. I couldn't help but think of my sister-in-law, Marcia and Billy, her husband, living for each CA-125 during her six years of survival with ovarian cancer. As my father used to say when he had to winter in Florida because of his health and I would join him for lunch sitting at poolside in his bathing suit playing pinochle; he would look at me and say, "Everything is called living!"

When I was out jogging that morning, I was thinking. Running was one of the best times to think. I was thinking of how we in the medical profession were using our senses less and less, and how having cancer seems to have heightened my awareness and made me a much better listener. Now I listen with all my senses it seems, much more so than before. I have always been amazed at how it is possible to listen and not hear. I watch my medical students and residents interact with patients and think how poorly they are using their senses and how often they are listening and not hearing. Well, I certainly don't think one needs to get cancer to start hearing. This reminds me of a patient I saw in our acute care medical clinic. This is a clinic that sees our regular patients or new patients making an initial visit or patients followed up from the emergency room or from other services, or after hospitalization. Usually a medical student or the intern assigned to the acute care clinic would see the patient first and then present the patient's history to me. However, there are times, for various reasons where I will just go in and see the patient myself. This was one of those times.

This particular patient was a woman in her early sixties who had made numerous visits to the acute care clinic and to the gastroenterology clinic for symptoms of a digestive disorder. After talking to her for a few minutes I was getting the feeling that I really didn't know what her problem was, that there was something going on I was unaware of. So I kept excusing myself and then coming back and talking some more. I told her several times that I wasn't sure I knew what her problem was, nor was I satisfied that the myriad of tests she had had, including endoscopy and CT scans, had given us an answer. When I entered her examining room for perhaps the fifth time she looked at me and I told her she looked like she was about to cry. It was only then that she told me she didn't want to bother me with her problems but that for the last nine months she had been struggling to make mortgage payments on her house because her house needed a new roof and, after paying for that, she was unable to meet her mortgage commitment. She was widowed, had no children and was about to lose her house. Now if that didn't give her heartburn and make food stick in her throat I don't know what would. She was frightened at losing her only asset and her home to boot. She had never told this to any of the other physicians who had cared for her. And she saw no way out. What was it that kept the physicians from getting to this vital piece of her history? Perhaps it is easier to order a lab test or get a CT scan or refer to a specialist than to sit and listen—and hear.

Let me give you another example. Julia G. is a 70-year-old woman I have been taking care of for the last five years. It was about that time she had her first episode of deep vein thrombosis, which made me worry about an occult malignancy. However her problem as it evolved was inflammatory bowel disease, ulcerative colitis. Her symptoms largely resolved with treatment and she was doing well without further flare-up on a milk-free diet and sulfasalazine, until several years later when she had a flare-up that refused to respond to asacol and prednisone. Finally, not knowing what else to do, I hospitalized her and allowed her gastroenterologist to direct care. With colonoscopy confirming activity of her inflammatory bowel disease and with very little response to additional treatment, she was discharged and referred to a surgeon for consideration of a colectomy.

Early in her hospital stay, I went to see her and sat next to her bed, more or less socially and simply let her talk. After only a few minutes she began to tell me about her brother and her husband who both had died within a few months of each other some five or six years before. Her sister-in-law had decided to have her husband (Julia's brother) cremated. Julia strongly disapproved, but she had no control. She did not go to Tampa, Florida, for the memorial service after the cremation. She never really forgave her sister-in-law. Recently her sister-in-law called her and wanted her husband's ashes buried in the family plot in Augusta. Julia, as the oldest surviving child, had legal control of the family plot and her sister-in-law had made arrangements for the burial before getting Julia's permission, and Julia was steaming about this, but only internally. Well, the burial service was to be the Saturday of Julia's hospitalization and Julia had told her sister-in-law she might still have to be in the hospital! Coincidence that her colitis was active? Did she need a colectomy? Or a confrontation with her sister-in-law? Or at the very least expressing her anger and coming to terms with her feelings? You tell me.

We arrived back home from Maine and Janet got on a plane the next day to go to Chicago to help our son Gary and daughter-in-law Lisa with their new 4 pound 13- ounce Alexis Nicole, born by C-section a week earlier. After one week taking care of their household while Lisa learned how to take care of and nurse a little baby, her first, Janet returned to me. It was good to have her back.

My first week back to work after vacation went well. I played tennis three times that week after work. I had finally returned to my pre-anti -androgen and radiation therapy weight. This was hard to believe, but my treatments had added 18 pounds to my weight and it had taken me this long to get back to my norm. My exercise and work pattern really had not changed much, nor had my diet, although it certainly changed because of the effect of the radiation on my digestive system, which made it difficult for me to eat my usual fruits and vegetables. I did eat more bread, which seemed to be a staple that did not upset my stomach, but my caloric intake was not a whole lot different. I also developed a real fat pad around my abdomen, as well as definite breast enlargement. I looked different, became more feminine in body habitus and had less muscle mass. This was all secondary to not having testosterone—again, something nobody told me would happen. I must admit that nobody but Janet saw me without clothes and therefore knew nothing of my breast enlargement or change in body habitus. As a matter of fact, Janet really didn't see me too much without my clothes. I was never shy with her before but I sure became self-conscious and made a real effort for her not to see me in broad daylight.

The other interesting thing that no one ever told me about was that I would smell different after radiation. For some time after the treatments I kept asking Janet if she smelled me and first thought it could be my perspiration. She never noticed anything. As time passed I began to realize that I smelled different, and not pleasantly so, after a bowel movement and when I was in the shower after a B.M. It then became obvious to me that what I was smelling was related to my defecation and this, in turn was associated with changes from radiation procto-colitis. This is not a big deal and by being extra careful, washing thoroughly after a B.M. it was never a big problem. You see, so much of what I went through and the complications thereof were not in and of themselves a big deal but they all added up. Not to realize these side effects was to be very shut off from myself and my feelings. But if all these things occurred to me and nobody warned me ahead of time, what about all the other cancer patients with far more side effects, and never forewarned?

You know, that reminds me of an experience I had years ago with a new patient in my office in Hollywood, Florida, when I was in private practice. I must admit I have always been very sensitive to odors. Sometimes I think it was because my kids were pot smokers and I developed a very keen sense of smell. I think I could smell marijuana if it was being smoked in the next county! Anyway, I always felt that a patient should be clean and neat when going for an examination to a physician. After all, I was always clean and neat out of respect for myself but also out of respect for my patients. I never enjoyed examining a patient with bad body odor. I mean not just unpleasant body odor but dirty, unclean body odor. It is not easy examining anyone in such circumstances, in a small examining room without windows.

There are very few times in my professional life where I ever told a patient to go home and take a bath, put on clean clothes and then come back. Such an event happened to me with the patient in Hollywood, Florida. He had absolutely terrible, insufferable body odor, and it was impossible for me to be in the small examining room with him without feeling like retching and without my eyes watering. My smeller told me this was just a dirty, unclean person. Rather than tell him, as I did not want to hurt his feelings, I spoke to his wife in private. She informed me that the odor was from his colostomy. You all know that a colostomy is a bag that collects feces in a patient who has been surgically deprived of a connection of the large intestine to the rectum. I did not for a minute think this was the case and the wife took her husband home and never returned. Now, so many years later, after experiencing the effects of my radiation on my post-defecation odor I wonder if I had been correct in attributing his bad body odor to being unclean.

Speaking of body odor reminds me of a college roommate I had for one semester at Oberlin. He had a severe case of hyperhydrosis. That is, his feet perspired excessively and the odor was unbearable. He was well aware of it but said there was nothing he could do about it. Our dorm room wasn't any bigger than the examining rooms in my office. Anyway, the minute I opened the door to enter the dorm room, if my roommate was there my eyes immediately began to water. Even after I acclimated to the odor, my eyes wouldn't stop watering. I could not read in my room and had to study in study halls and other friends' rooms. After one semester I had to change roommates out of self-preservation. Somehow these experiences conditioned me to be very sensitive about odors.

of New England Medical Center. What an exhilarating experience, having Ally with me at that time. We opened up the sofa bed and Jeff and Ally slept right next to our bed. Having Ally with me was like a breath of fresh air, a ray of sunshine, giving me the feeling that, perhaps, there was still a life for me. The next morning we four—Janet, Ally, Jeff and I—drove to our home in Friendship and had a most wonderful weekend. That Ally is something else. Okay, she is my grandchild, but she really is something else, something very special. There is such depth in her eyes, when she looks at me, and a warmth, an understanding, a connection that has nothing to do with her age—which was all of 16 months at the time.

Well, perhaps I felt the same when Ashley, my oldest grandchild, was two years old. It is wonderful to love, and to be loved. Because she is so special to me? When I see Ally, and see the look in her eyes when she looks at me, I feel a special glow. Her unfettered, unconditional love makes my spirits soar.

Dan Rahn told me at the very beginning of this cancer ordeal that I would need spirit, I really had no idea what he meant, but it did not take long for me to know exactly what he was talking about. I really do not know how he knew, but he did. It reminds me of the song from the Broadway show, "Damn Yankees":

You gotta have heart.

All you really need is heart.

And with cancer all you need is SPIRIT, in capital letters. Come to think of it, there is a real similarity there; that is, between having heart and having spirit. I really do not think anyone can get through cancer treatment

Chapter Fifteen

SPIRIT

This is at the heart of the matter—spirit. I was thinking about this when I was running in Westlake, Ohio. I was visiting my son, Jeff, his wife, Sharon, and my favorite granddaughter, Ally, (and baby sister, Abbey). This was August 2000 and Ally was two years old, and I admit we had a very special relationship, different from that with any of my other grandchildren. I know this had to do with the fact that Ally was with me in Atlanta for the weekend when she was eight months old, and I was attending a medical meeting a few days after finding out I had prostate cancer— and, more importantly, when I was at Tufts New England Medical Center in Boston for three months, getting radiation treatments for my prostate cancer.

Jeff had brought Ally up for the weekend. Janet and I picked them up at Logan Airport, and they stayed with us in our one-room residence at the Neely House without a whole lot of spirit. Without it, I think I would become seriously depressed and withdrawn and have to ask myself a thousand times, is it worth it? Not only that, your spouse needs to have spirit as well.

Let me tell you what I mean by spirit if I can. This is a bit difficult to define and I really never thought about it until Dan mentioned it. I do not think he was talking about religion. In teaching ethics to my medical students, I have tried to incorporate spirituality into my teachings. By this, I include religion but do not equate the two. For instance I believe an atheist can have spirituality and I believe a highly religious person may in actuality be devoid of spirituality. To me, Dan has both a committed, deeply religious conviction, as well as a deep sense of spirituality.

When Dan and I talk about spirit, it isn't religion we are talking about, but rather how one faces and deals with a life-threatening illness, one that does not kill immediately and suddenly; rather one that has stages: (1) diagnosis; (2) treatment—enduring it and its after effects (later I will talk about energy which is an integral part of how one traverses this rocky road); (3) remission, or that period of time after treatment and before the cancer re-emerges, if the cancer patient is fortunate enough to have a remission; (4) re-treatment and its effects and after-effects; (5) the terminal phase, with its physical and emotional challenges, including that of facing one's imminent demise.

I am in stage 3, I hope. I have survived stage 1 and stage 2, although I am still dealing with some side effects of treatment. But I am not complaining. My life goes on pretty much as it did before cancer. But, without question, there is an added dimension to my life just from having had cancer. I am still working full-time which, I must admit, takes not only spirit but energy as well; still jogging and working out daily; still playing tennis regularly; and still in love with my wife—and loving her physically when and if I can, which is not too often and not too macho, but to be able to do so is still a blessing.

Perhaps being where I am and doing what I am doing is what spirit really is.

I must, before closing, briefly mention my dear friend and companion, a quirky little yorkie-poo who found us shortly after we arrived in Augusta and stayed with us until his death from cancer in August 2004, four years after my treatment began. His full and final companionship during our parallel cancer experiences so vividly brings forth for me the enigma of life's ironies: the unexpected occurs; the sadness expands; living and dying continue.

I detail mine and Fred's "Race to the Finish" in Appendix II. I will only briefly tell you at this point, that, over the years that followed our meeting, we developed an intense friendship, based on mutual caring, understanding, trust, and that indefinable connection, or simpatico, that makes two people, or man and his dog for that matter, come together over time. We came to depend upon each other, to need each other, and yet learned to respect each other's privacy.

Fred's cancer first became apparent about one year after mine was diagnosed and initially treated. Suffice it to say that, after five surgical procedures to palliate his cancer, which began in his mouth and, after four years of watching and waiting, he succumbed. By 2003, Janet felt I would have to put him to sleep as his suffering continued to increase. And yet, as difficult as watching him suffer was, I didn't want to be without him. Isn't this the same dilemma we face in our own lives, and in our medical practice, and why we struggle so with the concepts of physician-assisted suicide and euthanasia? Ironically, we put our dearly beloved animals to sleep (i.e., active euthanasia) when we think it is in their best interest, and yet, to offer this to our dearly loved human relatives fills us with such uncertainty, indecision and angst.

By May 2004, Fred was in a lot of pain, in spite of analgesics, and Janet could not stand seeing him suffer this way, and wondered whether keeping him alive with such limited quality of life was fair. Still, he was my old buddy, my loyal friend. But the race, I feared, was nearing the finish line.

August 23, Fred was barking in a different way, awakening me at 3 a.m. By 7:30 a.m., he was barely able to stand, and could not eat. The tramadol and prednisone for pain relief just didn't help. He couldn't get away from his pain. We couldn't bear to see him suffer so. When I examined him I felt a large mass in his belly, and knew for certain, his cancer was metastatic and lethal. I knew today was different—Fred was dying.

I called his veterinarian, shaved his foreleg and injected a vein with Demerol. I had never done this before and didn't even know if Demerol worked for dogs. In fact, I didn't know if that amount, which I had used at times with my human patients would kill him, but didn't think at this point it would matter. Fortunately, it relieved his suffering, and we took him to Dr. Grayson Brown's office. In the car, on my lap he already seemed to be separating from us.

When we got to the office, we all realized Fred's time had come. He had lived a good life, but recently his life had been more an existence than a life with any quality. He had lived and loved and now it was time to end the suffering, end his dying process. It made me think of the designation "AND" that Chuck Meyer, a hospice chaplain, coined to replace the "DNR" or "Do Not Resuscitate" designation we currently use in medicine. AND means "allow a natural death." That is what we decided for Fred.

And so the race to the finish for Fred and me ended. I have to ask—did Fred win the race? Yes, he died first. Is that the victory? The answer may not be evident, but at least Fred's suffering has ended. Perhaps, in that sense, it is a victory. And now, in due time, I will follow him. I don't know when, but I do know it is just a matter of time.

EPILOGUE

February 2009

Can it be 10 years since my diagnosis of prostate cancer? My PSA is now 19, which is worrisome indeed. And yet, with interrupted therapy, my PSA was 20.14 in June 2006. What does it all mean? My cystoscopy yesterday revealed no recurrence of the bladder cancer, and so life seems to go on. How my prostate cancer was and is being treated is an example of how little we know of the natural history of this malignancy.

What, then, should one's philosophy of life be? I have my Janet and that is my philosophy, my raison d'être, my reason for wanting to stay alive. I do believe, as Langston Hughes once said, "Birthing is hard, and dying is mean—so get a little loving in between!."

There is no moral to this story. I only hope those with prostate cancer, and their loved ones, count each day a blessing and know that others share their sadness, their pain and suffering, and, yes, their happiness as well, during their journey with prostate cancer. I am there with you and, perhaps sometime, in the now, or the hereafter, we will meet and share our experiences.

Appendix I: further reading

For those who would like to read more on related topics, I offer these suggestions for further reading: titles that have helped me and may help others.

Nadine Jelsing, PROSTATE CANCER; PORTRAITS OF EMPOWERMENT, Westview Press (1999). In a retreat for prostate cancer survivors, 10 men discuss issues of concern: diagnosis; treatment choices; side effects; their health care team; living with prostate cancer; strategies for survival when recurrence occurs; and how their choices affected them and their partners and families. This is a useful reference for alerting prostate cancer sufferers to alternative medicine therapies.

David Biro, "MY ONE HUNDRED DAYS; MY UNEXPECTED JOURNEY FROM DOCTOR TO PATIENT, Pantheon Books (1997). A young physician with a life-threatening blood disorder called paroxysmal nocturnal hemoglobinuria describes his initial reactions to the first event that led to the diagnosis of PNH, and some of the issues that arise when a physician is also the patient. He gives a warm personal account of the involvement of wife, parents and sister. This is an informative look at having a life-saving bone marrow transplant and how two specialists disagreed on what was the best form of treatment for him. It is a candid account of the author's harrowing experiences as a patient, and how, ultimately, he was forced to decide for himself whether to have a bone marrow transplant or not. In this book, the author describes a short period of time in his life when he had to come to terms with a life-threatening illness and differing opinions as to how his illness should be treated, and he recounts his difficulty in deciding which treatment to accept.

Barbara Rubin Wainrib, Ed.D., and Sandra Hakers, Ph.D., with Jack Maquire, MEN, WOMEN AND PROSTATE CANCER, New Harbinger (2000). This is primarily addressed to the women who care for men during their illness with prostate cancer. It offers detailed, life-saving information about the condition and takes readers step by step from cause, detection and diagnosis through treatment, recovery and post-treatment life.

PROSTATE CANCER: A DOCTOR'S PERSONAL TRIUMPH, by Saralee Fine and Robert Fine; Paul S. Eriksson (1999). Radiologist Robert Fine and his wife, Saralee, tell the story of his prostate cancer and their quest for the right treatment. With his medical knowledge he sometimes knew almost too much. He received special care in being a physician, and eventually chose brachytherapy as his treatment modality. It is valuable as a resource for others with prostate cancer who do not have the type of access available to the Fines, nor the background to digest it.

HUMANIZING PROSTATE CANCER: A PHYSICIAN-PATIENT PERSPECTIVE, by Roger E. Schultz and Alex W. Oliver, Brandylane (1999). A urologist and one of his prostate cancer patients have combined perspectives in a book to help men and their families cope with prostate cancer. This interweaving of medical information from a urologist with the first-person account of a patient offers a rather broad perspective on how to better deal with the diagnosis of prostate cancer, the treatment options available and some of the emotions of the patient throughout the process. Families and patients will find this book informative and helpful in facing this illness with perhaps less fear and anxiety.

APPENDIX II: A RACE TO THE FINISH

Now is the winter of our discontent …
The Tragedy of King Richard the Third
Act 1, Scene 1
William Shakespeare

So it comes down to this: does Fred die first or do I? And how did it come down to this? Perhaps if I start at the beginning … . Janet and I moved from Hollywood, Florida, to Augusta, Georgia, 10 years ago. We moved into an old house set up on a hill, with the city reservoir behind us, an empty lot to the side of us and a large lawn and driveway running up to the house from the street below. Our living room faced the street side of the house and was surrounded by low azalea and lariope. It was the front part of the room that became Janet's music studio and it was here that she positioned her baby grand piano.

Shortly after moving in, Janet's sister, Marcia and her husband, Billy, arrived for the weekend. They were inveterate walkers, and one of their walks that weekend took them down Park Avenue, a shaded, divided, tree-lined street three or four blocks from our house. It was there they first encountered Fred, and it was in that encounter that Fred's destiny and mine became interwoven. For some reason, known only to Fred, he decided to follow them to our home. He never really left us after that, even though he never came into our house, nor was he ever restrained or tethered. In truth, there were very rare times when Fred was allowed indoors, and those times usually provoked by a lightning storm, which never failed to thoroughly terrify Fred.

He was a quirky little guy, funny looking, highly suspicious of humans, initially shying away from any human contact. He weighed all of 16 or 17 pounds, at most three hands high, with a mixture of shaggy black and brown hair, hanging from his parts in a most chaotic, disingenuous way; perky ears; a wagging tail; deep, expressive, brown eyes; and a totally whimsical, individual style and behavior. The first few weeks after he arrived, we mostly saw him sitting out front listening to Janet playing her piano, and sometimes joining in with a howling sound as he pointed his snout heavenward. It was a good few weeks before he would come close enough for us to offer food and drink, and even longer for him to accept. Eventually he did accept, and, in doing so, became part of our family.

The veterinarian, when first meeting Fred, told us he was a yorkie-poo, probably three to five years old, previously neutered, and seemingly quite healthy. His fear of humans, however led us to believe he had been abused. He had a habit, for instance, of turning in a circle, typically three times when approached, and this continued long after he accepted us as his adopted family.

If you have never seen a yorkie-poo (or Fred, *our yorkie-poo*), you are in for a good laugh. His personality, though, is purely Fred, and it is his behavior, in addition to those large, sad, and intelligent brown eyes, and his remarkable loyalty and affection, that make him so endearing.

Over the years that followed, Fred and I developed an intense friendship, based on mutual caring, understanding, trust, and that indefinable connection, or sympatico, that makes two people, or man and dog, for that matter, come together, over time. We came to depend upon each other, and to need each other, and yet learned to respect each other's privacy.

It wasn't until 1999, when my prostate biopsy revealed my highly aggressive prostate cancer, that our relationship began to change. For one thing, we had to leave Fred for three months when my cancer treatment necessitated our relocating to Tufts-New England Medical Center in Boston. We left him in the care of competent professional sitters as well as a dear friend, Betty Sussaman. Fred had lived outside independently, and, I believe, comfortably, but we had never left him for three months. As difficult as it was for me to leave him, I felt he would be better off in his own normal environment than trying to acclimate to a new place and new routine. Nevertheless, the separation was difficult, but Fred and I weathered the storm.

In our marriage, Janet and I discussed everything as honestly, candidly and openly as humanly possible. Our love sustained us, and only rarely did we find it necessary to hurt the other's feelings. And so with Fred it was so difficult for me not being able to talk to Fred, to tell him of my cancer, my changing life expectancy, my philosophy of life, his future and how much he meant to me. It is interesting how I used to consider myself a fatalist, as was my father before me. But my cancer made a believer of me and I no longer felt that what would be would be. No, I was suddenly frightened and far from ready to face my imminent demise. And as much as I wanted to share all of this with Fred, I knew it wasn't possible.

I returned home and, initially, my cancer seemed to be in remission. My PSA stayed below 1.0, and life went on pretty much as before. I continued to work full-time, to love Janet full-time, to jog and play competitive tennis regularly, and yet never, for one day, without anxiety about the return of my cancer, and my ultimate mortality. So Fred did not share knowledge of my cancer, the effects of the treatment I had received, or any awareness of my anxiety regarding my survival; not, that is, until early 2000, when I noticed the growth in Fred's right lower mouth. The growth was adjacent to his lower side teeth arising from the gingiva. It looked like a pink, tiny oval balloon with two smaller, satellite balloons attached. Fred didn't seem to mind having the lesion, but I certainly did. Cancer was not on a back burner in my thoughts, not at all.

The first biopsy was diagnosed as a sarcoma, which, in humans, at least, is a very serious connective tissue malignancy. The veterinarian had to put Fred asleep for the procedure and I worried about how Fred would handle such an insult. He was probably 12 or 13 years old by this time, although his exact age was unknown. In any case, he was not a kid, and he was certainly approaching old age, if not already there. Unfortunately the growth soon came back. The second surgical extirpation of the tumor returned a tissue diagnosis of amelanotic melanoma. This is an aggressive malignancy, often found in the oral cavity in male dogs, with a tendency to recur and to spread to the lungs. Fred continued to tolerate the tumor and the surgeries, seemingly going on just as I was going on. More than ever I wanted to converse with him, to share my misgivings of these veterinarians who never seemed to remove the tumor in toto. I knew only human medicine but my experience did not leave me well prepared to tolerate this incomplete tumor excision time after time. And so the tumor recurred and was removed three more times. It was only after the fourth excision that I noticed the vet hadn't removed the entire growth. When I discussed this with her, she informed me that she thought she had gotten it all and would be happy to see Fred and do further surgery. However, I elected to wait until the growth became bigger and more in Fred's way (or perhaps more in my way, as in became increasingly unsightly as it enlarged).

It was about the same time that my PSA took a big jump, signifying that my cancer was escaping from the effect of the radiotherapy treatments and hormonal manipulation I had received. In other words, I was considered at this point, a treatment failure. Ironically, Fred and I had reached a critical point in our lives, both faced with decisions to make, and each faced with the possibility of an imminent demise. I so wished that Fred and I could come to some meeting of the minds as to how to proceed; but Fred and I communicated in a far different way, and I could only try to imagine what Fred might have wanted, had he been able to tell me. Would he have wanted me to continue aggressive treatment, to go to great lengths to keep him alive no matter how poor a quality of life he might have? Or would he have wanted to forego such treatment and allow nature to take its course? Comfort care or continued aggressive care? Exercising what I considered to be reasonable substituted judgment, I made the decision for him. I made an appointment for him to be seen at the University of Georgia School of Veterinary Medicine in Athens, Georgia. In many ways, veterinary medicine is far less sophisticated and less technologically advanced than the medicine we practice as humans. In any case, they decided to do a wide excision and Fred survived the surgery in good shape. Much to my surprise, the path report this time wasn't melanoma or sarcoma but a nonmalignant, poorly differentiated, not well classified tumor! I wanted to believe this but, for one thing, I wondered how a nonmalignant tumor could be poorly differentiated! However, my naïvete led me to believe that academic veterinary medicine was far more competent and sophisticated than the family vet was capable of. Or perhaps I just wanted it to be so.

Still, at this point in time, Fred had a reprieve and I wished I could tell him so. No longer did it appear to be a race to the finish. My thoughts were, at this time, if old age doesn't get him he could well outlive me!

June 23, 2003

Fred's tumor continues to grow and I don't know how much longer he can go on. I know he is in pain at times because I can hear him crying. He stays under the hedges near my kitchen window and he cries, particularly after eating. If I give him half an Aspirin, he seems to get some relief. Yet when I come out in the morning, he is glad to see me, comes up to me with his tail wagging. His appetite remains good but he isn't all that comfortable eating. I see him at times trying to, very gingerly, get rid of the tumor with the side of his paw, but he barely touches the growth. It must just be too painful. The tumor is about the size of a small golf ball, and protrudes from his right lower mouth. It is ugly, ominous, and obviously painful. His spirit, however, remains good and, even when I go out after I hear him crying, he comes up to me as always, seemingly cheerful. I give him his aspirin in a spoonful of grape jelly and he takes it without difficulty. The tumor has not broken through the overlying skin but I worry that that is not far off. Janet thinks I will have to put him to sleep. Perhaps she is right. I cannot watch him suffer and still I don't want to be without Fred. Isn't this the same dilemma we face in our own lives, and why we struggle so with the concepts of physician-assisted suicide and euthanasia? Ironically, we put our dearly loved animals to sleep (ie: euthanasia) when we think it is in their best interest. Yet, to offer this to our dearly loved human relatives fills us with such uncertainty, indecision and angst. I understand this so well as I watch Fred with his tumor, and hear him cry, knowing it is just a matter of time until my hand will be forced.

As for me and my cancer, I have been on anti-androgen treatment for 19 months, following the biochemical post-radiation relapse. My PSA remains low, but three months ago went from 0.07 to 0.2. I wonder whether this is the beginning of the cancer cells becoming androgen-independent?

My next leuprolide injection is due in one month. I have decided not to take it. I do not want to live, knowing that as long as I take these shots I will never make love to Janet again. More than that, not having testosterone is an abomination. Not only can't I make love to my wife, but I really don't care. I cannot feel her, feel that feeling inside that makes me reach out to touch her, to want to be part of her physically when I see her brushing her hair, or preparing for bed. I must have my testosterone again. I will stop the leuprolide, track my PSA, and hope it will not rise so rapidly that treatment must be resumed. Not having libido sucks. What I live with now is the memory of what it was. I hate not having testosterone.

June 25, 2003

Fred was suffering but I wasn't convinced he was ready to die. The local veterinarian agreed to do a palliative surgical procedure. Again, my naïvete controlled the day and I allowed her to do another surgery. How could I have been so naïve? Yet, at this time, I was certainly not ready to put him to sleep, not convinced that there wasn't an aggressive, talented surgeon capable of helping Fred.

July 29, 2003

Hadn't this veterinarian been given ample opportunity to prove her competency? I guess human nature is to trust the caregiver you know, no matter what. After the surgery, it was obvious that little palliation had been accomplished. The tumor was still visible to the naked eye, albeit a little smaller, but obviously not completely excised. How could I have been so gullible?

We left Fred for three weeks with our housekeeper visiting and feeding him every day. We had a vacation planned and our home in Maine to go to. It was difficult leaving him, but again I felt it better to leave him in his own surroundings. He can barely see because of cataracts, his hearing is poor and he gets too nervous for even a short car ride, let alone a 1,300-mile trip with one overnight stopover.

I cried when I returned home—cried when I first saw Fred. I picked him up and he was just skin and bones. He was weak, tired, old, and had a tumor in the right side of his mouth that was bigger than before. One tooth seemed to be protruding from the tumor itself. There was tumor under his jaw as well, and it smelled. Ironically, the hair on his leg where he had been shaved to receive his intravenous for the June surgery hadn't as yet grown back. The growth of the tumor had certainly outraced the hair growth! I was sick with sadness and worry.

Perhaps having me with him again, or perhaps the spoon-feeding of soft food, or a combination of all, caused Fred to rally and he began to recover. His eyes were less glazed, his movements more certain, his tail began to wag, and he interacted with me as before. He still cried, however, after eating, even with the pain medicines I crushed and added to his food.

The tumor continued to grow, was terribly ugly to look at, and I did not think he could put up with it for much longer—nor could I. I knew we had to consider putting him to sleep, but I wasn't ready and I didn't think Fred was either. We scheduled a visit with another veterinarian who made house calls and she was no help, never suggested more surgery. She simply sent me information on squamous cell cancer in dogs, and a bottle of pain pills.

September 12, 2003
I knew there were no miracles but Fred was perky and more like himself except for the unsightly and inexorably enlarging growth. I couldn't accept euthanizing him, not yet.

My good friend, Bill Strong, took his dog, Molly, to Jim Wilkes. I decided to grasp at straws and ask a fourth vet for help in what seemed a futile endeavor. And so Fred and I visited Dr. Wilkes. Much to my surprise, he said his partner, Dr. Brown, was a skilful surgeon and might consider operating. He cleared it with Dr. Brown and we had an appointment one week later.

September 18, 2003
I liked Dr. Brown from the moment I met him. I liked his no-nonsense approach, his professionalism and his empathy. He understood the bond Fred and I shared and was willing to give Fred a chance, a last chance. Surgery was scheduled for the following morning.

September 19, 2003
I left Fred with Dr. Brown early in the morning and went on to work. About one hour later my pager

beeped. Dr. Brown was calling to tell me he had put Fred under anesthesia and opened the tumor site. He found the tumor wasn't encapsulated, and had gelatinous tentacles extending downward and backward. It would be difficult surgery, at best, and the outcome tenuous. He wanted to know if I wanted him to put Fred down. My reflexive response was clear and simple: No, I want Fred to have this last chance. Do the best you can. And so the surgery proceeded.

I arrived at the Martinez Animal Hospital late that afternoon. Dr. Brown met me and told me Fred was awake, eating, and alert. But he would keep him overnight because of a drain that was necessary in the operative site. It would stay in for 10 days, but the first 24 hours excessive drainage made caring for Fred at home difficult. And so I left Fred in their capable hands. For the first time with all of Fred's surgeries, I felt confident and that Fred was in the hands of a real doctor.

September 28, 2003

Fred's recovery thus far has been incredible. He no longer smells. I can pet him without his shying away. He is far more alert and more comfortable than he has been in months. His appetite is excellent. I can look at him and not see an ugly growth hanging from his lower mouth. He even barks at strange noises, a behavior that had been absent for a month. He stays out of his recent "home" in the bushes now, and often is laying near our back door, his favorite place over the years. In short, Fred has been given a reprieve. This wonderful, capable and courageous Dr. Brown, understanding my resolve, and Fred's being a survivor, gave Fred at least a chance at living yet another day. Thank you, God, for giving Dr. Brown his special gift.

October 23, 2003

My good friend Fred, is alive and well! He eats soft food twice a day and I no longer hear him crying during the day, or after eating. His vital functions are intact, his spirit is good, his mouth is well healed and, for now, I see no tumor residual. Life goes on for both Fred and me. Neither of us have signs of recurrent cancer. Yes, we both have cancer, and most likely, we will both die of our cancer, but for now we are alive and well. The race to the finish continues.

February 21, 2004

I cannot believe this happened but, when I pulled into my carport this noon and then turned around to park near the back door, I ran over Fred. Somehow, he didn't manage to get out of the way. I heard this terrible screaming. It took me some seconds to realize it was Fred. I was barely moving. When I stepped out of the car he was lying on his side under the car with the back of the left front tire pinning him down. I immediately backed away. I was certain I had killed him but he was able to get up and limp away from the car. How did this happen? For the last 12 years he has been outside and never did I think he wouldn't take care of himself. We have gone through so much together, and after getting a bit of a respite from his tumor, his good friend runs him over! I kept thinking: this is February, not the ides of March.

Janet wasn't home. I didn't know what to do. For him to have survived so much and then have this happen—I felt like a murderer. And, of my long-time friend yet.

Well, somehow, he was still alive. Janet called me and I told her what happened. She told me to call Dr. Brown. It was noon Saturday, but his office had him call me back. By now, 40 minutes later, Fred was limping badly but able to put weight on all four legs. I knew it was his left back leg. This was the one that bothered him in the cold weather. I felt his chest and abdomen, which he allowed me to do without evoking any pain. Dr. Brown said that it was probably a bad sprain and to give him Aspirin. And that is what I did.

It is inconceivable to me that I did this and that Fred actually was run over by me. Yes, he can barely see and, yes, he is nearly deaf, and yes, he is an old man, but never could I have imagined this happening. But somehow, it seems as if Fred has survived yet another insult, and this time at the hands of his trusted master and friend.

May 2, 2004

Fred is slowly but steadily losing ground. He cries a good deal and often can barely walk. At times he is so skittish, doesn't want to be touched, has trouble lying down, and so stands a great deal and eventually can lie down. I have been giving him Prednisone and Aspirin, which seems to help, but his breathing is more labored than usual. He is still eating, though, and usually wags his tail and is glad to see me. Janet cannot stand seeing him suffer this way and wonders whether keeping him alive with this quality of life is fair to him. Still, he is my old buddy, my loyal friend. He tries to look upbeat for me, but just doesn't make it. And yet, I cannot put him down—not yet. But the race, I fear, is nearing, the finish line.

June 30, 2004

Fred is crying—crying a lot. It seems worse after he eats and when he attempts to lie down. This business of lying down is a major problem for him. I watched him standing for what seems like hours before he tries to do so, and then the crying commences. It is quite unnerving, listening to him. I did take him to see Dr. Brown. He examined him and concluded that Fred was just a "decrepit old man" with arthritis and near blindness from cataracts and plain old age. So I give him Aspirin and Remadyl, which is like Vioxx, and an occasional Ativan.

July 26, 2004

My PSA is slowly rising. I am on no medicine now, but my anxiety level is rising with my PSA. This is what I refer to as "getting beat up my a number!" I know it is only a matter of time for me. Fred's time may be up before mine—only time will tell. In the meantime we are going to Hiawassee for a week on a Lake Chatuge, and must decide what will be best for Fred. We can no longer leave him to fend for himself while we are gone, and taking him with us would be too traumatic for him. So Dr. Brown will keep Fred in their kennel on Washington Road. They have asked me to send him with his food, a mat that he knows is his, and one of my old shirts or something to comfort him! Talk about caregiving. I just realized that is exactly what I have become—not Fred's friend, but his caregiver! Now that I think of it, Fred is like one of my patients: no longer able to make decisions for himself and dependent on a surrogate decision-maker and caregiver, a loving and loved family member, perhaps. So, in the final analysis, I must make decisions for Fred and care for him just as we must do with our loved family member.

Really, is an end-of-life situation for a dog and his master any different from that of a son and his dying father, in terms of decision-making, responsibility, and eventual outcome? What a lesson for medical students and young physicians; a parallel, perhaps, and a commonality with those end-of-life issues that they will face with their patients and families. The only difference is that Fred doesn't get to have any part in the decision-making process. Here, paternalism is not the exception but the rule. There is no advance directive; Fred has not told me anything about what he would have wanted in this situation, so there is no substituted judgment. There is only the best interest standard—that is, what would any dog in this situation be likely to want? Since we will never know the answer to that question, we must decide for our canine friends, and hope we make the right decision. But for now, I am not ready to put Fred down.

August 22, 2004
Fred is different today. At three this morning Fred was barking in a strange way. I can't tell you how different, just that his bark was different. I put him in the studio and he seemed able to rest. I went to get him out of the studio at 7:30 a.m. He was barely able to

walk, tail down, more or less limping, weak and not at all happy. He could not eat. He went into the bushes. I gave him Prednisone and some Tramadol, which is a pain medicine, but nothing helped. He just couldn't get away from his pain. He tried to go into the buses but kept barking this strange bark—something between a bark and a cry and whine. He only stopped when he saw me or when I patted him. This went on for four hours. Janet and I could not bear to hear him and see him in so much pain. I examined him. He now had a tumor growing from the left lower jaw whereas previously the tumor had been on the right. In addition, he had a sausage-like mass in his right abdomen. It wasn't tender but a mass for sure, and quite large. And so, Fred's tumor must indeed be malignant and now metastatic. Whatever, I knew today was different. I knew Fred was dying.

I had to do something. I called his veterinarian, Grayson Brown. While waiting for him to return my call, I shaved Fred's right front leg, and, with Janet holding him, I was able to find a vein and give him 50 mg of Demerol. I had never done this before and didn't even know if Demerol worked for dogs. In fact, I didn't know whether that amount would kill him, but didn't think at this point it mattered. Fortunately, he was able to get comfortable with the Demerol. Dr. Brown called me back and told us to bring Fred to his office. Janet drove and I held Fred in my lap, thanking God that at least he was not in severe pain. But it seemed like he was already separating from us. He offered no resistance, and seemed almost indifferent. When we got to Dr. Brown's office he and his wife comforted us. We all realized Fred's time had come. He had lived a good life and recently his life had been more an existence than a life with any quality. He had lived and loved and now it was time to end the suffering, end his dying process. It made me think of the designation AND that Chuck Meyer, a hospice chaplain, coined to replace the DNR designation we currently use in medicine. AND means, allow a natural death. That is what we decided for Fred.

And so the race to the finish had ended. I have to ask—did Fred win the race? Yes, he died first. Is that a victory? The answer may not be evident, but at least Fred's suffering has ended. Perhaps in that sense it is victory. And now, in due time, I will follow him. I don't know when, but I do know it is just a matter of time.

APPENDIX III: MOM

When my mother died at the Medical College of Georgia Hospital several years ago, I thought that, as a practicing internist of over 30 years, an associate professor of medicine at an academic medical center, and the creator and chair of the ethics curriculum at the Medical College of Georgia, I thought I was well prepared for my mother's final illness, perfectly confident in knowing not only what my mother wanted, but having her advance directive as well. How wrong I was! Not only was I uncertain what to do, but I realized that all of my training meant not a thing in helping me make that final decision. And no one was able to help me. For this reason, and for all those family members facing and making similar decisions for their dying loved ones, I dedicate this story, and I want you to know I know how difficult this can be.

Mom died at 1:40 a.m., March 15, in her hospital room on the sixth floor of the Medical College of Georgia Hospital. She was receiving nasal oxygen, intravenous fluid, and intravenous morphine, which I administered when necessary to keep her "comfortable." I am not at all certain she would have considered herself comfortable, even with the morphine. Perhaps the word, morphine, made us, who were with her while she was dying, more comfortable. My wife, Janet, and I were with her, and had dozed off. For some inexplicable reason, we both abruptly awakened at the moment of her last breath, as if we sensed her death. Perhaps the silence of her not breathing anymore was what we heard. I think it was more than that. At that moment of death both Janet and I felt we could see her soul leave her body, see her soul rise heavenward. We talked about this later, and both had the same sense of this departure.

The last four hours of her life were peaceful. The 16 hours before that were awful.

Mom was 92 years old and never the same after she had been found on the floor of her kitchen six months earlier. We never found out what happened to her that night, but what I knew was that her persona, her self, if you will, was gone. What she had been was replaced by a shell of her former self—a body who ate, drank, slept, and even answered questions, but offered nothing spontaneously. She seemed to have lost all initiative, or curiosity, or the ability to interrelate as she had before.

When Janet and I realized she wasn't improving, we moved her from Florida to an apartment in Augusta and furnished it with all her furniture, so as to make it as close to what it had been like in her previous apartment. We hired round-the-clock caregivers, and were able to see her several times a day.

At first, she showed very little improvement, but gradually, her appetite improved, she proceeded to gain weight, and was able to ambulate with a walker. Still, the Pauline everyone new, never returned. Her interest in her world seemed markedly blunted, but yet her face would light up when we arrived, as if she hadn't seen us in a long, long time. She thus became an enjoyable part of our everyday lives, as we became of hers.

The months were marked by subtle signs of progress, then new setbacks. Another fall strained her back. Then she fell and sprained her ankle. Most intriguing to me was that, when she hurt her ankle, she insisted on calling me. Whatever my mom didn't know, she knew that she had a son—her son the doctor! This was literally the first time since her original fall that she expressed initiative of any kind, her first self-initiated phone call in six months.

Three weeks before her death, mom became agitated and displeased with her caregiver one evening. This was a remarkable change. It was as if Mom had returned. She became so much more aware of her surroundings; she started asking questions, and interacting in a way she had not been capable of before. Mom was back and we were thrilled.

Then a respiratory illness set in motion her final decline. We weren't ready for this to happen. I wonder if anyone ever is. Yes, we had her advance directive, and knew that she hadn't wanted to be on life support for a catastrophic illness. And yet we were tortured by the fact that perhaps this was a self-limited illness from which she could recover with assisted ventilation. We decided to honor her directive.

This was, for me, one of the most difficult decisions I have ever made. She was, at this time, still alert, but too ill to communicate in a meaningful way. Janet and I knew how much she was suffering, and her eyes seemed to be asking, "Why aren't you doing something for me?" And I wondered whether we shouldn't be doing something more. Were we making the right decision? Didn't Mom deserve one attempt at bronchoscopy and assisted ventilation? There was no question she would die without it.

Janet and I, at her bedside in the emergency room, agonized over this. My years of practicing medicine, and teaching medical ethics, all of a sudden mattered not a whit. It was as if I knew nothing of living wills, autonomy, and medical decision-making. I was now only a son who wasn't ready to lose his mother.

Nothing seemed real, except seeing Mom fight to breathe, fight to stay alive. This became unbearable. I suctioned her myself, frequently, to ease her discomfort, and perhaps to ease mine. I was, after all, her son, the doctor.

And so I watched her die. Not being able to do something for my mother when she needed me most was excruciatingly painful. I felt as if I was not there for her when she needed me most.

After Mom died, I continued to agonize. Would she, facing death from an incidental, albeit catastrophic event, have wanted heroic measures in spite of her advance directive? Perhaps there are no answers. My medical knowledge and experience didn't help me. I was left with one overwhelming emotion: I watched my mother die and I could not help her.

If there is a lesson to be learned from this experience, it is that a greater force exists than our finite, limited one. Too often we cannot influence the process of life and death. This, then, is my lesson. And as the pain of Mom's death lessens with time, her legacy is her memory. I will always remember her smile and pleasure when she saw me. I will always remember the last four months of her life, of what we shared, and the joy of her life when she was once again close to us. And, someday, when the pain and grief of losing her diminishes, I will be able to accept the fact that I did all I could, and that my mother rests easy, knowing this to be true.